WHAT YOU SHO
FROM Uꭒꞇꝺ

Learning to Live with Undifferentiated

Connective Tissue Disease

Kimberly McBee

WHAT YOU SHOULD EXPECT FROM UCTD

Copyright 2014 by Kimberly McBee

Cover Design, William McBee

Website: http://www.kimberlymcbee.com

ISBN 9781494766733

DEDICATION

This book is dedicated to UCTD. Without you, I would not be who I am today. As you wrecked my life, you created new pathways.

To my husband William who was fortunate every night to have to listen to pages of this book. He was also lucky enough to have to design this book cover. I thank him for his support and dedication.

To my parents Joycelyn & Daniel, this unforgiving disease has shown me the depths of your love.

To my baby sis Kerry, you have fed me, held me and dried many a tear. Blessings and prosperity be yours.

For everyone else who provided support, I thank you.

TABLE OF CONTENTS

PREFACE

Hello, my name is Kimberly McBee and I have firsthand experience with the challenges of having UCTD. I wrote this book to provide an insight into diagnosing, recognizing the symptoms and managing the UCTD disease.

Discover why it is so difficult to get diagnosed with UCTD. Learn what to expect from doctors and the available treatments available for your UCTD issues. Explore alternative therapies and coping techniques and explore available treatment options.

This book highlights the challenges, the triumphs, the frustrations and the uncertainty of the UCTD journey. In addition to over 110 content pages on the disease, this book also has 70 current medically available reference links on the UCTD disease.

The information in this book is not meant to be medical advice. Please consult with your doctor before embarking on any new medical or non-medical intervention. Please do not to use information from this book without consulting your doctor. This book is not meant to provide a cure or exclude medical care. The statements in this book unless otherwise noted, have not been evaluated by the FDA. At the time of publication, the reference links provided were active links.

« CHAPTER 1: THE DISEASE »

I have UCTD, the invisible illness. I often joke that this disease is so invisible that some doctors are not even aware of it. For years, I thought I did not have a real diagnosis and kept trying to obtain a "correct" diagnosis. Now I know better and have redirected my efforts to learning more about this disease and educating others.

Trying to explain to others that I had undifferentiated connective tissue disease has been no easy task. Many persons have never heard of it and seem to think it is a "made up" disease. To the contrary, this disease is very real and currently wreaks havoc in my life and the lives of millions around the world. In this book I will explore the disease in all it facets and intertwine my personal journey with this illness.

Undifferentiated connective tissue disease (UCTD) is indeed a confusing disease. While accepted by some doctors as being a real illness, it has been rubbished by a few who think the disease is all in the patient's head. According to Dr. Jessica Berman[1], the term "undifferentiated" in UCTD simply indicates that patients have not "differentiated" into having well-defined connective tissue diseases (CTD) issues. Nonetheless, UCTD patients do share connective tissue issues and should be treated accordingly.

UCTD might be termed as the lesser known cousin of well-known connective tissue diseases such as Systemic Lupus

Erythematosus (Lupus), Polymyostis & Dermatomyostis, Sjögren's (SS), Scleroderma and Rheumatoid Arthritis (RA). Connective tissues in the body include the skin, cartilage and other joint and organ tissues. CTD issues occur when the body's connective tissue is attacked by the body's immune system.

In normal persons, the body's immune system is designed to repel bacteria and other foreign invaders that may cause infections and illnesses. However, in patients with UCTD and other connective tissue disorders, the body's immune system mistakenly views the body's connective tissue as a foreign invader.

UCTD patients experience autoimmune issues caused by the body's constant fight against itself[2]. The term autoimmune refers to issues with the immune system where autoimmune issues result in connective tissue diseases. In a compromised body, the body's immune system attacks otherwise healthy connective tissue causing pain and suffering to the patient.

In my first visit to my rheumatologist (rheumy), he employed allegory to explain my autoimmune issues. He explained that the immune system was made up of little soldiers marching around the body. At certain points, and without obvious reason, these soldiers would stop and attack the joint tissues thinking that those tissues were actually the enemy. As such, my rheumy explained that this is what caused my low grade fever, joint pains and swellings. Who knew that a war was occurring daily in my body? I certainly I didn't.

Patients with UCTD share some similar symptoms and general health issues as persons with well-defined CTD; however, the UCTD patients might not fulfil all the established criteria for one of the connective tissue diseases[3]. My rheumy was probably initially concerned that I had lupus as my symptoms were closest to a lupus designation. However, while I had many of the lupus symptoms I did not fit the clinical or diagnostic profile for lupus. Consequently, given my symptoms and blood test results, my rheumy decided to diagnose me with UCTD, meaning I had connective tissue problems but had not differentiated into a well-defined CTD disease.

Over a decade after becoming ill, I have not differentiated into a well-defined connective tissue disease, neither have my symptoms disappeared. According to accepted literature, within the first year, some patients differentiate into well-defined connective tissue diseases like Lupus while others remain undifferentiated.

Some patients do see an improvement in their symptoms over time and might even recover. Other patients like myself, have to live with UCTD and are termed to have stable UCTD. Such patients will have periods when the disease seem to be in remission and other periods when such patients experience flares of disease activity[4].

In some cases, you might hear of someone having MCTD or mixed connective tissue disease. This is not the same as UCTD as MCTD patients do have more than one well-defined connective tissue diseases. MCTD therefore refers to patients who manifest symptoms of multiple connective tissue diseases. These patients can then be clinically diagnosed with an overlap syndrome. Thus a MCTD patient could have Lupus and another CTD at the same time with symptoms indicative of both diseases; hence the term 'overlap syndrome'[5].

Autoimmune & Inflammation

The term autoimmune does not refer to one specific disease. There exists an entire group of diseases classified as autoimmune of which UCTD is only one such disease. It is difficult for a lay person to identify autoimmune diseases solely by name as many of the diseases do not have the term autoimmune as part of their name.

These autoimmune diseases are often systemic and affecting the connective tissues of the body or organ-specific where only certain organs are affected. What all these diseases have in common however, is that they are all drivers of inflammation.

Much of the discussion around CTDs involves inflammation. Inflammation is the key driver of our autoimmune issues and is sometimes difficult to manage. A 2011 PubMed Health article[6] highlighted that inflammation is "the body's immune systems' response to stimulus." When you are injured, your body tries to heal itself and revert to its previous healthy state. In repairing the injured area, inflammation causes more blood and defense cells to reach the area of injury. Hormones are then released to inform the brain that the injury has occurred; prompting our attention to the injury. As a result, the injured area may often pain (the signal that something is wrong), have an elevated temperature and swell in response to the healing process underway.

White blood cells[7] or leukocytes as they are known are responsible for defending the body against infection and viruses. Lymphocytes are particular types of leukocytes responsible for blocking all harmful antigens. These harmful antigens include but are not limited to viruses, bacteria, damaged cells and foreign tissue. The immune system creates B cell and T cell lymphocytes to fight the antigens; however, these cells sometimes also attack healthy tissue.

Many persons might be more familiar with the idea of the body's immune system producing antibodies to fight germ and viral threats to the body. While each of us has naturally occurring autoantibodies[8], the problem occurs when the body sometimes mistakenly produces too many antinuclear antibodies (ANA). These antinuclear antibodies are responsible for attacking the nucleus of your cells thus causing havoc with your immune system.

Testing for these antinuclear antibodies is one way to detect the presence of an autoimmune disease. In my experience, some doctors put too much emphasis solely on the results of the blood tests. For more than one doctor, I was determined to be well as I did not have high levels of ANA.

Please note that not having high levels of ANA does not mean you do not have an autoimmune disease. Similarly, having high levels of ANA does not mean you have an autoimmune condition as persons can have high levels of ANA but be healthy. As the blood test is only one way of diagnosing an autoimmune condition, do not allow a doctor to rubbish your concerns simply because the blood work showed normal levels of ANA.

As a result of the immune system constantly waging war against the body, chronic inflammation may occur. Chronic inflammation or systemic inflammation occurs when the body tries to repair what wasn't injured. As such, the immune system is called on to fight phantom foreign invaders (bacteria & viruses) to the body. Having not found the expected infection, the immune system still mistakenly fights and this creates high levels of unwanted inflammation in the body. High levels of sustained inflammation will result in chronic inflammation and have deleterious effects on the body.

According to PubMed Health, at the site of the inflammation, manifested symptoms might include one or a combination of swelling, redness, elevated temperature, pain and loss of function of the area. Typically the body reacts to inflammation with an elevated body temperature, fatigue and a general feeling of malaise. These reactions should be familiar to CTD patients as they most likely experience those feelings of fatigue, feeling unwell and suffer from chronic low-grade fever.

An Allegorical Example of our Immune System

The 2001 movie Osmosis Jones provided a lighthearted view of what happens in response to viruses entering the body. The titled character Osmosis (Ozzie), a leukocyte, lives in a host body. His job is to help prevent bacteria and viruses from entering and causing havoc in the body. Ozzie however, mistakenly reacted to a perceived virus and caused a negative bodily reaction to occur in the host body. Here, you might recognize that our immune systems cause us the same grief. Our misguided immune systems are currently the bane of our existence as they produce inflammatory responses to phantom or perceived threats.

Later in the movie, Ozzie triggers a cramp in the host's leg while pursuing other viruses. This scene also resonates with me as I can attest to this happening when I am sick. I sometimes have those unexplained muscle cramps in my calf. Now I know who to blame! My allegory concludes with Ozzie receiving help from Dix who is a suppression medication. Together they try to neutralize the invaders in the body and return the body to full health. Isn't this the same great ending we would all like? Finding medication that works with and for us?

My UCTD – A Journey to Wellness

I remember the first time I started having joint issues in year 2000. I was living in the UK and my ankle had started swelling frequently and would pain me terribly. A visit to the doctor confirmed that the swelling was due to the impending winter and the fact that my tropical Jamaican body was trying to adapt to a new climate. Six months later, and a second doctor's visit provided me with no new clues. Instead, the doctor surmised that I simply needed to stand less.

Two years later, on returning to Jamaica, I began feeling exceptionally fatigued. Persons tried telling me that it was natural to feel tired. However, I could not accurately convey that there was a vast difference between feeling very tired and having the constant feeling of exhaustion. Finally, one mid-week morning, I could hear all happening around me but I could not get up to get ready for work. I could not summon the energy to even call out for assistance. Finally, someone came into the room to check why I wasn't up for work and realized that I wasn't well.

At the time, I was living in Kingston, Jamaica and I remember clearly, my mom having to drive 30 miles to Kingston in order to take me to a doctor. The years that followed my initial episode included numerous doctor visits, trying new medicines, trying new foods and alternative therapies. At times I have become increasingly frustrated as the years revealed no new research on the disease and no cure in sight.

I can emphatically state that you too might have to search for years before you find the optimal formula for getting well. Do not get discouraged; keep reaching for your goal of good health and feeling well.

Identifying the Causes

UCTD occurs when the body's immune systems mistakenly attacks the body's tissue. Although the exact cause in unknown, the good news is that UCTD rarely results in tissue and organ damage. An article in The National Institute of Health noted that up to 22 million Americans suffer from an autoimmune illness.

While UCTD can occur in anyone, it is most likely to present in women between the ages of 30 and 50 years. According to Fairweather and Rose (2004)[9], women are disproportionately affected by autoimmune issues with as much as 78% of autoimmune sufferers being females. Fairweather and Rose further posited that over 80 diseases are directly or indirectly caused by immune issues.

Persistent research into the cause of many autoimmune diseases has yielded little more than hypotheses. UCTD therefore, remains an autoimmune condition of unknown origin. However, it has been hypothesized that the disease like other autoimmune diseases might be a result of environmental exposure, viral infections or even genetic predisposition[10].

UCTD environmental triggers might include toxins and stress. Both these triggers are possible causes of autoimmune issues although a direct link has yet to be established. Exposure to mercury or mercury poisoning is a suspected cause of autoimmune issues. For example, persons with amalgam mercury dental fillings are said to be at increased risk of mercury poisoning and subsequent health issues. Additionally, improperly disposed mercury discharge ends up into streams, rivers and seas where fish like salmon and tuna are affected.

If you doubt that mercury is hazardous, consider that it is because of mercury concerns that pregnant women are warned to avoid sushi and other dishes containing certain fish. Mercury has been found to affect the unborn fetus. Mercury is particularly alarmingly to some homeopathic practitioners who warn that mercury affects the body's tissues and causes changes to the tissues. You will remember that our immune systems will attack anything that it perceives as a foreign invader. Thus, if mercury affect our tissues, causing changes, it is not inconceivable that our immune systems will attack those tissues.

Mercury is not the only environmental toxin affecting our health. Years ago, I watched a documentary that showed the level of heavy metals present in the soil, our waterways and even our drinking water. These heavy metals are said to be damaging to our adrenal system and overburdens our liver. If our liver is working inefficiently, then our hormone functions may be affected and our body's immune system thrown into chaos.

Stress is also an important consideration when trying to identify causes of autoimmune issues. Stress can wreak havoc on the body and may be the precursor of some autoimmune conditions. Stress is known to affect the immune system and some persons report experiencing severe stress prior to becoming ill. There has yet to be strong statistical results showing stress as a cause of autoimmune conditions. The fact the stress occurs in the life of an autoimmune patient does not necessarily make it causative.

Aside from stress, infections are another likely cause of autoimmune diseases. While I cannot remember having any major infection prior to my diagnosis with UCTD, some persons do report having viral infections prior to exhibiting symptoms of UCTD. For some, they remain unaware that they have an underlying infection that is causing their health issues.

Among connective tissue disease sufferers, two common underlying viruses that often remain undiagnosed are Lyme and Epstein Barr. In support groups I have been in, I noted that quite a few persons reported discovering that they had gone undiagnosed with Lyme or Epstein Barr. Consequently, it is advisable to exclude the possibility of having these viruses.

Apart from viruses and toxins, genetics is said to be a contributory factor in autoimmune conditions. For some, there is no genetic link that they are aware of. Personally, I have had a family member die from lupus related issues and first cousins that suffer from multiple sclerosis (MS) and myalgic encephalomyelitis (ME). In recent years, I have heard my sister complain about increasing joint pains and other symptoms that I recognize as my initial symptoms of UCTD. Whether or not those symptoms develop (and I hope they never), it does seem that there might be at least a possible genetic link.

Much has been mentioned in recent years, about the quality of our food being a factor in the increase in autoimmune illnesses. Some physicians and homeopaths posit that autoimmune conditions can be reversed or improved by changing diet and lifestyle. For some UCTD sufferers, food allergens are the basis of their illness and a change in diet will most certainly positively impact their health.

In most accepted UCTD literature, food allergy is not given as a possible cause of the illness. This does not mean however that a food allergy is to be dismissed. Further in this book I discuss illnesses caused by food allergies and how diet can impact your overall health.

Recognizing the Symptoms

UCTD symptoms vary for each person; develop at different stages and result in varying levels of pain and discomfort[11]. No two person's story might be alike, but a general pattern may be seen among persons suffering with UCTD.

Fatigue – this is not your normal feeling of being occasionally tired. This feeling of fatigue will be persistent and impact your daily life. Some doctors recommend making time in the afternoon to have a short recharging nap to bolster your energy levels and enable you to complete your day. For some patients, the fatigue will be debilitating and prevent them from carrying out many normal functions in their homes or work.

Fatigue was one of my main symptoms and it caused worrying issues such as affecting my ability to drive and maintain full-time employment. My level of exhaustion would be so severe that I would stop in mid-sentence and my eyes would begin closing. At that point, only a quick nap could rejuvenate me and I would be ready to continue what I was doing prior.

Headaches – persons may or may not have been troubled with headaches prior to developing UCTD. What is sure is that the type of headache, the frequency and the intensity of headaches may increase.

Neuropathy – Peripheral neuropathy[12] may result in feelings of numbness and pain, burning and a sense of weakness in hands and feet. Peripheral neuropathy can occur outside of the extremities and impact other areas such as your stomach causing gastrointestinal issues. Neuropathy is related to the nerves in the body that transmit signals around the body; these signals originate from the brain and spinal cord.

Initially when I became ill, I was constantly tested for diabetes. These numerous diabetes tests were to rule out the neuropathic issues I was experiencing in my fingers and toes. I would get tingling sensations, pins and needles as well as localized pain seemingly shooting from my finger tips and my toes. With diabetes suspicions dismissed, the doctor could then concentrate on other diseases that included symptoms of neuropathy.

Vision problems – the inflammation which is such a large characteristic of UCTD affects all parts of the body, including the eyes[13]. UCTD vision problems are also sometimes caused as a side effect to medications such as Plaquenil; a commonly prescribed UCTD drug known to cause potential vision issues.

I am unsure as to what caused or is causing my vision issues as I have been on drugs that affect the vision over time. As such, I advocate that you ensure that you are checked yearly by an ophthalmologist to ensure that your vision problems are addressed. I speak more on the need to regularly schedule ophthalmologist visits in chapter 3.

Low Grade Fever – temperature occurring between 99.8° F-100.8° F is considered low-grade fever[14] . Low grade fever is an indication that something wrong is happening within the body. In the case of UCTD, high or rising levels of inflammation in the body can cause low grade fever.

For years, each morning I would wake up freezing cold. The cold would be so extreme in my bones that it would wake me from deep sleep. As much as I lived in Jamaica, I would have to keep a comforter on the bed in addition to my sheet. And at times, even that would not be enough to keep me warm. Additionally, some mornings I felt feverish and would fight to get warm only to "sweat out" the fever a hour or so after the episode first began.

Joint pain & swelling – arthralgia occurs when your joints hurt and can be mild or severe. At the place where two joints meet (knees, elbows, ankles); patients with UCTD may experience soreness, pain and swelling[15]. In some cases, sometimes your joints may also feel warm to the touch and the joint may have low grade temperature.

I am a human barometric pressure gauge. My joints can predict rain way before I see the first rain cloud. My joint pains intensify around certain thunderstorms, thankfully not all. I am finding that colder temperatures do not translate into increased joint pain as some would believe but does result in increased swelling in my legs.

Weight loss/weight gain – weight loss is a possible symptom of UCTD, especially when coupled with other symptoms listed. Surprisingly though, persons with UCTD might actually experience weight gain as sometimes they have been prescribed medication for what doctors think is another illness. Such medications such as antidepressants might cause weight gain.

Alopecia – hair loss befalls some UCTD sufferers. Women are sometimes the first to realize their thinning hair and subsequent hair loss. For some sufferers, the hair loss is very apparent when they try to wash their hair and the hair falls out in clumps. In some cases, overlapping autoimmune skin conditions can also cause alopecia.

Ulcers – mouth ulcers are common symptoms of UCTD. UCTD sufferers report numerous instances of mouth ulcers that may even interfere with eating or drinking. For some patients, nose ulcers also occur and can be quite painful.

Dryness of mouth and eyes – eyes may be gritty and itchy and it may become difficult to produce tears thus necessitating eye drops. Dry mouth and insufficient saliva production is another issue, one that can lead to tooth decay if not addressed.

Frequent colds & infections – given the compromised immune system of the patient, the patient is more likely to experience frequent colds and infections. I had multiple infections in the first few months of becoming ill and the doctors could not figure out why I was so susceptible to getting colds.

Sensitivity to heat and the sun – the heat of the sun and photosensitivity to sunlight and some bright UV lights can cause great discomfort for UCTD sufferers. The sunlight can actually feel painful on the skin and in some cases a rash may develop after being in the sun. The sun also exacerbates fatigue and creates a sense of malaise.

Heat and direct sunlight often has debilitating effects on me. Something as simple as shopping in an outdoor farmer's market is enough to send me to bed the next day. No matter my energy level before the shopping outing, by the end of the outing, I am always left feeling extremely fatigued and sometimes a sense of feeling sick to the stomach.

Raynaud's (cold affects hands and feet) – this phenomena causes the fingers and the toes to become almost as cold as ice and to turn blue in some cases. The extremities including the nose and ears may become extra sensitive to cold temperatures because of limited circulation to those areas.

Abnormal nailfold capillaries also occur in tandem with Raynaud's and is one of the clinical diagnostic criteria for secondary Raynauds. Doctors test for abnormal nailfold capillaries patterns by microscopically observing the patient's nailfold changes over time.

Pleuritis or pericarditis – this happens rarely but occurs when the inflamed lining around both the lungs and heart which result in chest pain when patients breathe. Also may cause shortness of breath.

Skin issues - some diseases manifest as skin conditions such as the butterfly rash for lupus or other skin rashes and thickening around the fingers and toes. Some persons may also experience scaly and inflamed patches of skin.

Lymph node swelling – your lymph nodes under your armpits, by your groin and your neck may become swollen and hurt when touched. Swollen lymph nodes are the body's way of indicating that something is wrong in your body. In the early days of my illness, my lymph nodes were so swollen that the doctors suspected my body was fighting an infection although they could not figure out what my body was fighting.

Muscle weakness – the muscle weakness could be prominent in one area or present in all muscles. Your muscle weakness could be mild to extreme where you are unable to maintain movement using those muscles. Muscle weakness may be indicated in your ability to do exercise, do chores or carry out your function at work.

17

As I write this book I am experiencing consecutive days of debilitating muscle weakness in my hands. On days such as this, it is a challenge to even lift my hands to comb my hair. These are the days when I find it difficult to open the door or to grasp a glass or a plate. On these days I have been known to lose my grip on breakable items. Yes, these are the days when the stores love me- those days when I break stuff and have to replace them.

Standing is also a major issue when my muscles are weak. My legs will literally begin to tremble and shake if I stand for extended periods of time. After 20 minutes standing in one place, my legs begin to feel weak and then begin to tremble involuntarily. It is good that I am not a dancer as after only a few moves, it is as if my legs begin yielding and I find I must sit or risk falling over.

My UCTD – Chronicling my Symptoms

My first symptoms were joint swelling and pain in my ankles. It would be almost two years later before I started noticing joint pains in my knees along with extreme fatigue. With this debilitating fatigue, I found that I would rest all weekend and yet be exhausted on Monday morning. Additional sleep or increased vitamin intake did nothing to alleviate my exhaustion. The more I pushed through the never-ending tiredness, the worse I felt.

During 2001 to 2002, I found myself getting a cold multiple times per month. It was also almost like I had a constant low grade fever. The doctors at this point simply kept trying to treat the simpler manifestation such as the cold but would ignore the other symptoms I noted. One doctor condescendingly told me that the flu "hurts" as a response to my queries about the constant fatigue and joint pains.

It was about this time that I also started noticing that my skin was hurting when I went in the sun. I remember being in the car and the heat of the sun was so intense that I had to move to the back seat of the car and lay across the floor of the car to try and escape the rays of the sun. Every spot that the heat of the sun touched felt as if it was on fire. I am glad that that symptom disappeared but occasionally my mom will remind me of that day and we reminisce on how ridiculous it was for a grown woman to be hiding from the sun.

By late 2002 to early 2003, I started realizing that even a light touch would hurt and by late 2003, I was having all over joint pains. I remember clearly that Radian-B muscle rub, an anti-inflammatory topical cream, became my new 'perfume'. The pain in those early days was relentless. Unfortunately, regular nonsteroidal anti-inflammatory drugs (NSAIDs) reduced but did not eliminate the pain and swelling. I remember my older sister Shirley stopping by on more than one occasion and helping me rub my joints when the pain got to be too much.

About this same period, I began having the most excruciating headaches and it became commonplace for me to be ensconced in my room. My room at this point was always kept pitch black to minimize my light-sensitive headaches. My headaches increased in frequency and intensity and prescriptions like Topamax did little to alleviate the severity of the migraines. Driving one evening, I was blindsided by one of these headaches and had to pull off to the side of the road and call someone to pick me up as I felt unable to safely drive any further. I certainly do not miss these headaches.

During all of these emerging symptoms, I kept visiting doctors to find the root cause. I was convinced that there was one explanation for all my symptoms but the doctors I saw chose to focus on individual symptoms. Personally, I feel that if I had a doctor who had considered my symptoms en bloc, I might have found relief much earlier than I did.

The symptoms soon impacted my career. As a teacher, I had started forgetting my lesson content. I remember crying one day as I could not remember the definition or examples of a pronoun. Additional cognitive challenges included forgetting the route I took to arrive at a location or arriving at a destination that I had not intended to visit that day.

I also began noticing that my reaction time and reflexes were not as sharp as were to be expected. To this day, I am unsure how these challenges all fit in with UCTD or if it was the beginning of the overlapping Fibromyalgia diagnosis I would get almost 7 years later.

As the disease progressed, I stopped driving as my fingers hurt to the point that I could not bend them to grip the steering wheel. Furthermore, my hands and feet would get so cold that they would hurt. It became evident that the environmental temperature was not the trigger. My extremities would be ice cold regardless of Jamaica's tropical 90 degree heat. In order to get some relief, I would have to immerse my hands and feet in warm water.

It was also about this time that I started to get body chills, and again, it was a strange sight to see me in the middle of a hot tropical day in a sweater: I could go nowhere without one. The chills would be worse in the mornings as would the exhaustion, and by this time in my illness, I felt I was out of options as no doctor could tell me what was wrong.

If I thought the symptoms were through, I was sadly mistaken. I soon started having shortness of breath in the middle of a conversation and even during singing a song at church. I must explain that it was not a hyperventilating kind of shortness of breath, but just a feeling that you needed to catch a breath. I am not sure when this symptom disappeared; although I believe it was after a period of taking my least favorite steroid- prednisone.

In recent years, I have enjoyed better health even though the symptoms have not ceased. I have experienced lessened intensity and frequency with my symptoms. However, do not get comfortable with this disease. Just when you think you cleared a hurdle, you may be unpleasantly reminded that this disease is unpredictable. Over a decade after the initial symptoms, it is still a bit frustrating to be discovering new symptoms. I try to remain upbeat and maintain a positive outlook. I encourage you to do the same and do not be discouraged.

If my story mirrors your experience, a frank discussion with a caring doctor can help you address how to mitigate your symptoms. Do not be afraid to change your doctor for one that will listen. Please note that symptoms might disappear or lessen through the use of medications, diet modification, exercise and alternative therapies, but the same results are not guaranteed for each person.

Flares & Remissions

As a UCTD sufferer you will most likely experience flares; periods when your symptoms are most exacerbated. Common treatment during a flare includes using corticosteroids such as prednisone as a means of suppressing the overactive immune system. The severity of the flare differs with each individual. Nonetheless, it is usual to see multiple symptoms intensifying in severity during the flare. The length of the flare varies with each individual and could be as little as a few days to as long as several weeks.

For me during a flare, it is like every joint remembers to hurt at once, my vision changes, my cognitive function diminishes and my Raynaud's shifts into overdrive. I have yet to figure out what triggers a flare as the situation before the flare and the time of year the flare occurs shows no clear similarities.

There will also be periods of remission, those happy days when you forget that you have an illness as you are asymptomatic. Remission to some might be that the disease managed while on medication. Thus the UCTD sufferer experiences no symptoms of the disease. However, most persons wish for remission while on no medication. This remission means that the disease is quiet and the patient experiences no symptoms.

For some UCTD patients remission may be temporary, lasting weeks or months while for others, the remission is prolonged and lasting years. Such lasting remissions is akin to the patient getting better and is the single most desired state to a UCTD patient.

I have yet to discover why remissions occur but I do enjoy and look forward to these times of remission. I must caution however, that overdoing it during this remission period may actually lead into a flare. Believe me, I have done it. I got so excited that I was well that I once again started working full-time. I also started a part-time business and began studying for my master's degree. Unfortunately, these ambitious activities soon resulted in my body "crashing" and I experienced a severe flare. A few weeks on prednisone did however help to shorten my recovery time.

Some persons were quick to note that I became ill because I overdid it. At that time, I disagreed with their observation. If healthy persons could do it and I was no longer sick, then why couldn't I do it too? Obviously my thought process was faulty, but my failure to maintain a regular life has not dampened my desire to be well.

At some point in this journey I learnt it was better to stop comparing my present life to my life before UCTD. My current goal is to discover what triggers my periods of remission so that I can replicate the conditions leading to an absence of my symptoms. See if you too can recognize what practices result in you having periods of remission

Pregnancy & UCTD

Having UCTD does not necessarily preclude your from experiencing motherhood. If you have UCTD, you can still try to have a baby. Like my rheumatologist, your doctor will want to run certain tests to ensure that your pregnancy goes well. I explain more on one blood tests in chapter 2. My primary care doctor recommended seeing a high-risk ob-gyn if I decided to get pregnant. She believes that the high-risk ob-gyn would be best suited to dealing with issues that might arise due to my UCTD.

Some women do worry that UCTD will severely affect their pregnancies and they worry about flares during what is already a stressful period. Anecdotally, I have read of women who report periods of remission during and immediately after their pregnancies. As such, please note that it is possible to have a disease-free pregnancy or experience minimum symptoms during your pregnancy.

However, I must note that some women might unfortunately experience a flare during their pregnancy. A very small percentage might even progress into a full connective tissue disease. Despite this, the prognosis for getting pregnant, carrying the baby to term and remaining well during pregnancy seems possible. Unfortunately for us, we can never predict which one of us will pull the short straw and become more ill as a result of being pregnant.

« CHAPTER 2: WHAT'S WRONG? »

According to Mosca, Tani, Carli and Bombardieri (2012, p. 73, ¶1)[16]:

The existence of systemic autoimmune diseases not fulfilling classification criteria for defined CTDs is a common clinical experience. These conditions have been variably defined as incomplete lupus erythematosus, early undifferentiated connective tissue diseases and undifferentiated connective tissue diseases (UCTDs).

Diagnosing UCTD

Patients having symptoms of a connective tissue disease, but who do not fulfil the clinical criteria for a defined CTD disease may be diagnosed with UCTD. Additionally, a positive result on ANA blood tests (more on this later in the chapter) can also be used to classify the patient as having UCTD. Even in the absence of positive immune markers blood test results, a doctor can still diagnose the patient as having UCTD especially if the patient responds to conventional medications used for CTDs.

Some diseases share similar symptoms with UCTD and as such, your doctor will request x-rays, laboratory tests and employ clinical diagnosis to rule out the usual suspects that might mimic UCTD issues. In the rest of this chapter, I examine commonly explored diseases and blood tests that might be necessary for your doctor to identify your underlying health issue.

The diseases and blood tests given in this chapter are not exhaustive or meant to be the total list; rather, they offer the most basic expectations you might ask your doctor to test against. For more information on these and other diseases, visit the National Institutes of Health's MedLine Plus website.

Connective Tissue Diseases Mimicking UCTD

Arthritic diseases occur when the body's immune system attacks itself. The similarity between the symptoms of UCTD and common arthritic diseases such as lupus, scleroderma, RA and Sjogren's syndrome, means that doctors must carefully exclude these diseases in order to diagnose UCTD. A doctor will normally order certain blood tests and check you against criteria for the different arthritic diseases.

Even though I tested negative for arthritic diseases, I seemed to have the symptoms most closely aligned to lupus. I remember one doctor watching to see if I would develop the lupus malar rash as I had been showing sensitivity to sunlight. The good thing about not testing positive for the major arthritic conditions is that the doctor can then focus on other diseases or known issues that may be causing your problem.

The autoimmune connective tissue diseases listed below share common symptoms that include joint pain and swelling, fatigue, headaches, low grade fever and shortness of breath amongst others[17].

Systemic Lupus Erythematosus (Lupus)

Lupus is more common in women than men and occurs at a higher rate of incidence in black women than the females of any other race. With lupus, the skin and the joints become affected by inflammation and major organ involvement often occurs. Unlike UCTD, if untreated, lupus may cause death. Lupus symptoms include a butterfly rash on the face, organ failure, sensitivity to light, memory and cognitive issues as well as joint pain and swelling.

Lupus does not have a cure but is managed by medication. The unfortunate thing is that a lupus diagnosis sometimes takes years. The length of time it takes to get a lupus diagnosis can severely impact the quality and timeliness of care.

Scleroderma

If you are woman of childbearing age then you are more than 15 times likely than men to get the disease. Less than 500,000 persons in the US have the disease[18]. Scleroderma affects the skin and organs as well as the blood vessels. Symptoms of scleroderma include thickening of the skin, gastrointestinal issues and Raynaud's phenomena.

Rheumatoid Arthritis

Inflamed joints and joint swellings are key symptoms with RA. The joints may become so stiff and inflamed that the sufferer loses mobility of that joint. RA affects the joint lining and over time, may lead to deformity of the joint. Other symptoms displayed are organ involvement, fatigue and weight loss.

Sjorgen's Disease

Eyes and mouth moisture glands are affected and the patient is bothered by dry and itchy eyes and a lack of saliva. Furthermore, fatigue and issues with the joint are also indicators of this disease. Sjogren sufferers must be aware that they are increased risk of lymphoma (cancer) as well as will most likely experience organ involvement and gastrointestinal issues.

Polymyostis & Dermatomyostis

These diseases are primarily characterized by muscle issues[19]. Muscle weakness may be mild to severe and is the most common complaint. Basic impairment may include difficulty in movement but can be as severe as difficulty in breathing. Other symptoms include Raynaud's phenomena, weight loss and fatigue.

Polymyostis and dermatomyostis are part of the group of diseases referred to as inflammatory myopathies. Unlike polymyostis, dermatomyostis also includes skin involvement such as a skin rash. Part of the testing process for these diseases includes a recommended muscle biopsy and your doctor may also test you to determine your muscle strength.

Other Diseases Mimicking UCTD

Multiple Sclerosis (MS)

This autoimmune disease affects the nervous system. The brain and the spinal cord are affected and the nerve signal between the brain and the body deteriorates and causes issues for the patient. MS can be mild but may develop to a serious condition where the patient is unable to walk or speak Common symptoms include muscle weakness, vision problems, concentration issues and trouble with coordination. There is no single blood test for MS and the disease is currently not curable although it is managed by medication.

My cousin in the UK has MS and is currently experiencing difficulties with walking. I sometimes wonder if there is any truth to autoimmune issues being a part of the family tree. Perhaps it is simply coincidence.

Lyme Disease

Lyme disease is spread by deer ticks that transfer the disease to humans through tick bites. Ticks are often found in outdoors areas and so persons must take care when camping or hiking. Lyme disease is treatable but the diagnosis is sometimes difficult as the doctor might not initially consider Lyme disease. Ensure that your doctor conducts testing for Lyme disease so that the disease can be ruled out. Symptoms of Lyme disease that mimic UCTD are fatigue, joint pains and neurological problems[20].

Sickle Cell Anemia

Insufficient healthy red blood cells in a person's body make it difficult to get oxygen around the body. With sickle cell anemia the red blood cells resemble sickles or crescents instead of the round shape of healthy red blood cells[21]. These abnormal blood cells are rigid instead of flexible and so get stuck in small blood vessels and prevent normal oxygen flow to the parts of the body. Persons with sickle cell undergo periods of body pain, swelling, fevers and vision problems which are similar issues UCTD patients' experience.

Crohn's Disease

Crohn's is the chronic inflammation of the end of the small bowel into the beginning of the colon. The entire gastrointestinal tract might be affected with diarrhea, constipation and abdominal cramps being major gastrointestinal symptoms. Other Crohn's symptoms that mimic UCTD include weight loss, fatigue and fever[22].

Celiac Disease & Non-Celiac Sensitivity

In some persons, gluten triggers their autoimmune responses. Celiac disease affects more than 2.5 million Americans and has led to changes in how food companies make and market foods. What for some is a normal meal might cause intense pain and damage to the body of a person suffering from celiac disease. So much of the foods we eat contain gluten in some form. Gluten is found in wheat, rye and barley products although some persons with celiac report issues eating oats or other grains that contact with wheat products.

The autoimmune responses that are triggered when a person eats gluten occur in the small intestine. Over time, repeatedly eating gluten can result in damage the lining of the small intestine[23]. Similarity in symptoms to UCTD includes headaches, joint pain and exhaustion.

Thyroid

When the thyroid gland produces too little hormones a person is said to be hypothyroid. On the other hand when the thyroid produces too much of the hormone, the person is said to be hyperthyroid. The thyroid gland controls most of the metabolic processes in the body[24]. Symptoms of hypothyroid include joint pain and swelling, memory issues and fatigue[25]. Hyperthyroid on the other hand has symptoms such as sensitivity to heat, fatigue and muscle weakness[26].

When I first became ill, I was constantly tested for thyroid problems as some of my issues mimicked thyroid issues. I remember my first tests results being what the doctor called borderline hypothyroid, however he didn't think that was enough to pursue the thyroid angle. Subsequent tests have not revealed any thyroid issues and so that as excluded from the continuing investigation into my health issues.

Interestingly, I have heard at least three anecdotal stories about persons having undiagnosed thyroid issues that were misdiagnosed or ignored. Consequently, ensure that your doctor conducts the appropriate tests to both identify and treat potential thyroid problems or to exclude thyroid issues as the basis of your health problems.

Chronic Fatigue Syndrome (CFS) & Fibromyalgia (FMS)

According to The John Hopkins Lupus Centre, in some cases, persons with autoimmune conditions also develop other illnesses or comorbidities such as FMS or Thyroid issues[27]. These other illnesses happen in tandem with the autoimmune condition and can sometimes make it more difficult to treat the exact cause of the symptoms. One of the issues I have had over the years is identifying which symptoms are UCTD and which are FMS. Obviously, correct identification of symptoms can lead to proper diagnosis and treatment.

Both CFS and FMS have long been debated as to their authenticity as bonafide illnesses. Some medical personnel once believed, and in my experience, some still do believe that patients are solely psychosomatic and thus should not be classified as being physically ill. Both CFS and FMS are sometimes seen as "garbage can" diagnoses, as they both are labels given to patients when the doctor cannot find anything else wrong with the patients[28].

CFS is largely defined by extreme fatigue but can include muscle pain, brain fog and insomnia[29]. FMS or fibro causes sensitivity to temperature, widespread body pain and involves pain and muscle weakness in the joints and muscles. FMS sufferers like CFS sufferers also complain about extreme fatigue and disturbed sleep patterns[30]. Memory and cognition issues are also major issues for some FMS sufferers and the term fibro fog was coined to explain the memory and concentration challenges FMS sufferers' experience[31].

The similarities of the symptoms with CFS, FMS and UCTD highlight how easy it is for a patient to be misdiagnosed. In some cases, doctors like my rheumy might diagnose UCTD with FMS depending on the symptoms exhibited by the patient.

Stress

Stress may not be a disease but is a precursor to many diseases and health issues. I include stress in this section as stress can cause numerous symptoms that can mimic UCTD and other connective tissues diseases. Over 43% of adults in the USA have health issues related to stress[32]. Symptoms of stress include gastrointestinal problems, asthma, skin conditions, headaches, sleep issues, back pain, difficulty concentrating and depression. Is it any wonder then that doctors are so quick to tell you that your multiple issues are stress-related?

Do not be quick to dismiss a doctor when they ask you about your stressors. Some of your symptoms could be stress related and may be eliminated by using some of the coping strategies in chapter 5. If you however believe that you have a genuine health issue and you are not stressed more than normal then find a doctor that is willing to listen to your concerns.

Blood Tests for Autoimmune Markers

Outside of the blood tests to identify the specific diseases discussed above, no single test[33] exists to identify autoimmune diseases and so multiple tests are conducted to give a clearer picture of what is happening in the patient's body. UCTD sufferers like other CTD patients will most likely do blood tests to check for:

Antinuclear Antibodies (ANA)

The ANA test is an indicator of the levels of autoantibodies in the body. Higher rates of these antinuclear antibodies may be an indicator of autoimmune issues. However, healthy persons may still have high levels of antinuclear antibodies and not have autoimmune issues. As such, this test cannot be the sole definitive measure for determining neither the type of illness nor the severity of an autoimmune illness[34].

As a part of the UCTD diagnosis, your doctor may conduct ANA testing at intervals over the course of three years. If you test positive for ANA on at least two occasions that may be one way of the doctor giving you a diagnosis of UCTD. Because UCTD is sometimes ever evolving, the long duration preceding diagnosis occurs because the as the disease changes, so might the results of your ANA test.

Some doctors seem to use the ANA test almost like a gold standard of testing. The pattern of the ANA test helps the doctor differentiate between the different autoimmune conditions and even specifies the type of a particular disease.

High erythrocyte sedimentation rate (ESR)

ESR is an indicator of inflammation in the body. High rates of ESR means that the levels of inflammation in the body are high and the patients is likely to be undergoing symptoms such as joint pains among others. ESR cannot be used to diagnose a CTD but is used to measure disease progression[35].

Presence of antiphospholipid antibodies

These antibodies are found in some CTD patients and can lead to miscarriages and premature births in pregnant women[36]. The antibodies also prevent proper blood clotting. My rheumy told me that this test was ultra-important if I was considering having a child. His concern was that if my level of the antibodies was high, it might indicate problems carrying a baby to term.

Markers of autoimmune disease

Common blood tests for the various autoimmune conditions include Anti-dsDNA (double-stranded DNA) antibodies, anti-RNP, rheumatoid factor (RF), anti-Ku antibodies anti-Ro/SSA and anti-SM (Smith) tests. These markers allow doctors to narrow which autoimmune disease they are dealing with.

For example the RF test indicates the rheumatoid factor antibody present in the blood and is especially indicative of persons who have or will develop rheumatoid arthritis (RA). Please remember that healthy persons can still present with this antibody as well as person with other auto immune conditions apart from RA.

« CHAPTER 3: THE DOCTOR IS IN »

Your journey to health will require you to visit numerous doctors including primary care physicians (PCPs), rheumatologists (rheumy), ophthalmologist, neurologists, endocrinologists and gastroenterologist. My best medical care has been under the care of a wonderful rheumatologist who takes care of my joint and muscle issues. He is not always able to handle my full range of symptoms and so I need to visit other specialists.

What Type of Doctor Do You Need to See?

I currently see an ophthalmologist for my deteriorating vision issues and recently, my ophthalmologist recommended me to a neurologist for further testing. The neurologist will handle all issues relating to my neuropathic symptoms including burning pains in fingers and toes and issues with my changing vision. It is worth noting that a good PCP is important as I was able to ask my PCP for a second opinion on the neurologist visit. My PCP did concur with my ophthalmologist and recommended I set up an appointment in short order.

In some cases UCTD patients will have gastrointestinal issues and issues with their endocrine system. I have yet to visit a gastroenterologist although I was referred by my dentist. At that point in my life, I was simply tired of doctors. I was tired of being prodded and poked and with no real answers at the end of the visit. Regarding my visit to an endocrinologist, I consider that a waste of my time and money. The particular doctor lacked bedside manners and did not seem interested in discovering my issue. I have yet to be back and subsequently, did not visit any other endocrinologists.

Below, I give a brief synopsis of the function of each doctor that you are likely to see. I believe that you should become familiar with the type of doctors that will handle your illness. With a deeper understanding of the role of each doctor, the better informed you will be in choosing the right health practitioner. Below I discuss the different types of doctors that you will encounter and the reasons why these types of doctors are important.

Primary Care Physicians

I believe PCPs' are your first line defense in maintaining your care. It is always easier to visit your PCP than to have regular visits with your rheumy. I recommend having copies of your blood work and any x-rays or other tests to share with your PCPs. For one, this reduces the likelihood of spending money to re-do tests and it keeps both your PCPs and rheumy on the same page.

My PCP follows the medication guideline of my rheumy. She will adapt my medication dosage as needed depending on my emerging or decreasing symptoms. Developing a relationship with a PCP is vital to me, as my rheumy visits are three to four months in-between. Consequently, I need access to PCP doctor in the event that I have new pressing health issues in that interim period.

When my vision issues first began, my PCP was the one to recommend an ophthalmologist to handle my eye problems. In another instance, severe back pains prompted my PCP to refer me to the orthopedic doctor who ended up diagnosing me with FMS (fibromyalgia). I am grateful to my PCP for the referral. The orthopedic doctor was better able to address my back pains and spasms as well as provide a diagnosis and suitable treatment plan.

It is therefore important to create a good working relationship with your local PCP so that your entire health issues can be managed and where necessary, suitable referrals made.

Ophthalmologists

An ophthalmologist is "both physician and surgeon" (¶1)[37]. Many UCTD patients have eye issues which might require the services of the ophthalmologist. In some cases, medications such as Plaquenil are known to affect vision. Consequently, regular eye testing is required while on these medications. The ophthalmologist can also work closely with your neurologist or rheumatologist especially where inflammation or neurological issues are the cause of your vision problems.

After taking one of the highly recommended FMS drugs on the market in addition to a popular anti-inflammatory drug, I woke one morning to find my vision severely blurred. This blurred vision lasted for two to three days with my eyesight never returning to its pre-existing state. I visited two ophthalmologists but as my vision was constantly changing, it ended up being months later before my vision had settled enough for me to get glasses.

One of the ophthalmologists had noted that the muscle of my eye seemed inflamed and recommended a dose of steroids and an MRI. The other ophthalmologist concurred that it was possible that the inflammation was the cause. She however hypothesized that chemically induced myopia was more likely the reason for my recent blurred vision and subsequent near sightedness.

With newly prescribed glasses to correct my vision issues, I thought my vision problem were over. However, just 13 months later, my vision issues resurfaced and this time, my ophthalmologist recommended visiting a neurologist. The hope was that the neurologist would better explain my changing vision. The journey to that answer continues.

Neurologists

Neurologists are important in your journey to health as they help to explain issues arising from muscle weakness as well as any other neurological complaint that the UCTD patient might have. I find it helpful to call ahead before my visit and ensure that the neurologist has experience dealing with UCTD patients. The doctor's understanding of UCTD helps to reduce the amount of time between recognizing and treating symptoms.

UCTD patients sometimes present with multiple overlapping diseases and as such, when common issues relating to the nerves and the muscles arise[38], the neurologist should be the obvious choice. With tingling and numbness in my fingers and toes and in the absence of diabetes or other illness that could explain it, I was referred to a neurologist. My impression was that she did not understand the underlying illness and so her remedy was a dose of steroids instead of a deeper investigation. Subsequent to this visit, I began ensuring that all specialist visits required a doctor who had at least basic knowledge of UCTD issues.

Rheumatologists

These are doctors best suited to handling your autoimmune issues. Rheumatologists are experts in dealing with rheumatic and arthritic diseases[39]. Your rheumy is a trove of knowledge of all things autoimmune and can recommend suitable treatment plans to help you get well. A rheumatologist not only deals with the physical ailments of the UCTD patient, but also deals with the mental issues arising from having UCTD.

My rheumy is great at providing alternative therapies and coping skills for dealing with UCTD. I find that he listens when I say I want to be on the lowest dose of medication. He gets it when I refuse to take some pills due to the potential side effects. He understands that while I need pain pills, I will never finish a month's supply as I only take pain pills when the pain is severe. As a result, he understands that he does not have a pill seeking patient and I would like to believe that impacts the way he treats me.

Gastroenterologists

Gastrointestinal issues seem to be a part of our goodies bag of symptoms. While your PCP doctor can treat basic gastrointestinal problems, the gastroenterologist is the best person to evaluate, diagnose and treat your symptoms. A gastroenterologist is considered a doctor of internal medicine and is trained to deal with disorders of the stomach, small and large intestines, esophagus, liver, pancreas and gall bladder.

If you suffer from repeat issues with acid reflux, then the gastroenterologist may offer you the best management of the condition. Usually, your PCP will refer you to the gastroenterologist when the condition becomes chronic and is not helped by commonly prescribed medication. In other cases, if your PCP cannot identify the problem then a referral to a gastroenterologist is necessary.

Endocrinologists

Like the gastroenterologist, the endocrinologist is a doctor of internal medicine. This doctor is responsible for illness relating to the endocrine system. The endocrine system is responsible for hormones. Hormones are necessary to regulate growth, reproduction, mood, metabolism and sexual function. These hormones are secreted by glands. Some of these glands include the Hypothalamus, Thyroid, Adrenal, Pituitary, Thymus and the Ovaries.

I visited an endocrinologist on the recommendation of my homeopathic doctor who had theorized that my adrenal glands weren't functioning. The homeopath thought that my extreme exhaustion was caused by adrenal failure. The endocrinologist disagreed with the homeopathic doctor but could not provide any solid clues as to what was causing my issues. I made two visits to the endocrinologist and was not impressed by the service level received. Instead of returning, I have my PCP order my hormone tests when necessary.

Choosing the Best Doctor for You

Overall, through the journey to wellness, it is possible that you will encounter one of the following types of doctors indicated below. Hopefully you will find the Saint early on in your search for relief. However, it is most likely that you will have to deal with a few of the other types of doctors listed below before finding the Saint.

The Saints

Those doctors who actually listen to their patients are really saints to persons suffering from UCTD. These doctors seem to be in the minority and it took me years to find one. Search for a good PCP and rheumy willing to spend more than 10-15 minutes with you. This illness is not the common cold and a simple fix is not in your future. As such, you must get good medical care and the Saint is one of your best options for treating your complete set of symptoms.

My rheumatologist is my Saint. In the absence of conclusive blood tests, he still opted to treat me based on my symptoms. Regarding the symptoms, he believed that if it walked like a duck and quacked like a duck then it was a duck and he would treat it as such. This approach was the best approach a doctor had taken in over 5 years since becoming ill. A mere six months later, after taking methotrexate and the other medications he prescribed, I was well enough to go back to work. Coincidentally or not, I have never been as sick as I was before my initial visit to him.

The Kooks

One doctor drew a picture of my head and explained that less than 2% of the population had an illness that could explain my condition and I was NOT in that 2%. He then went on to explain how positive thinking could cure me. Of course his remedy was anti-depressants and the recommendation that I avoid stress.

44

Another doctor tried to hug me and then started asking about my personal life. Is your father in your life? Do you have a boyfriend? Do you have children? He then decided that I was a 28 year old who probably had baby fever and it was affecting me as such. Did I mention I went to see him for producing milk although I had never been pregnant? Probably I should also note that he did not touch me or examine my breasts to verify or rubbish my claim. I still wonder why I paid him.

A private hospital that I visited for outpatient services had a doctor who spent a long time with me. After visiting so many quacks who had not taken the time to listen, I felt so honored that he was taking the time to chronicle the issues and how they were changing. Imagine my surprise on my next visit when I realized that there was no record of my symptoms. It seems that the doctor in question had simply humored me; and had recommended a psychiatrist, as he believed I had too many seemingly unrelated symptoms. Funny enough, I did go to a psychiatrist who recommended me to see a doctor as the issue seemed to be genuinely related to the body.

The Prescription Writer

This doctor loves to write a prescription even though he or she cannot or will not tell you what is wrong. The first time I was prescribed steroids; the neurologist prescribing did not, or could not adequately explain the reason behind prescribing me prednisone. Other doctors have written numerous prescriptions for anti-depressants as easily as sending me to buy candy. I finally got fed up and told one doctor that with the amount of anti-depressants I had been prescribed and tried, I should have been well by that time.

The prescription writers are sometimes the ones to also quickly tell you that all your symptoms are psychological and are caused by stress. In my experience, stress is the go-to answer when doctors cannot tell you what is wrong. Note to doctors, not every issue requires an anti-depressant and not everything is simply stress.

It is possible that your health issue could be psychosomatic (of the mind) and exacerbated by stress. However, in my experience and from other anecdotal stories, years of suffering have sometimes revealed underlying health issues and proof that in some cases, the issues were somatic (physical) all along. The sad thing is, in seeking to pin a psychological label, some doctors leave us patients untreated for years and inevitably cause us more pain and suffering over time.

The I-Know-More-Than-You Doctors

Sigh, this is one of the worst doctors to encounter. I remember telling one that my not being a doctor did not denote a lack of intelligence, but rather spoke to a career choice outside of medicine. These doctors sometimes present as a KOOK as they try to show you the patient just how much they know and you do not.

This doctor either never explains things in simple terms, preferring to use the most scientific language possible or oversimplifies to the point of talking down to you. The positive is that this doctor is normally brilliant and if he or she took the time could probably have solved your problem. Unfortunately however, this doctor is more inclined to hear him or herself speak.

The Why-Do-I-Still-Practice Doctors

A doctor fell asleep while listening to my symptoms. If you do not have UCTD or another connective tissue disease, you might wonder why it would take longer than 5 seconds to list your symptoms. However, most connective disease sufferers do have multiple overlapping symptoms and must ensure that the doctor is aware of each one. Each symptom could be the difference between remaining undiagnosed and finally getting the care you need as a patient.

Another doctor gave me Panadol for pain despite the fact that stronger pain pills like Vimovo and Arcoxia minimized but did not stop the pain. It seems that most of his medicines were from yesteryear. His prescription read like 'what I would have prescribed in 1990' versus what 'I need to prescribe in 2005.' Taking pills that do not help you means adding unnecessary toxicity to your body without good reason. Personally, I do not advocate for taking unnecessary pills especially when those pills do not bring relief.

As a patient, you must ensure that the medications that you receive from the doctor are relevant to the time you are living in. I have called back a doctor and requested an updated prescription and I did not pay for it. Do not get brow beaten in paying for additional visits because a doctor did not take the time or apply common sense in prescribing your medication.

The I-Do-Not-Care Doctors

These doctors will make you feel like you are bothering them. Their tone is curt and their bedside manner leaves a lot to be desired. A prominent doctor on the island once prescribed a drug that had I known what the drug was, I would never have taken it. In defense of the pharmacist who filled the prescription, he did pull me aside and ask me if I was sure I wanted to fill the prescription and at that strength. Foolish me, I thought that if the "great doctor" prescribed it then it must be good.

Fast forward two or three days and I am crying uncontrollably (my nieces who were about 6 years old at the time still remember). Turns out that the pill was an anti-depressant/anti-psychotic and I had a bad reaction to it as I do with ALL anti-depressants. My mom called the doctor and his response was almost a shrug of the shoulder- 'it should have worked and if it didn't then I do not know." That was the end of his involvement as he felt he had done enough to try to help me.

Trust your Judgment

Sometimes you know that your doctor is not a good-fit. You sense the level of disinterest coming from your doctor. You might have recognized the unnecessary testing you are required to undergo, but you decided to stay silent. Does your doctor seem vested in you and your health challenges? If not, exercise your options. Find a doctor who cares, one who listens. I have heard that finding the right doctor feels like coming home. I know that feeling, and would love you to experience it too.

Medications

For UCTD patients, the road to recovery is a difficult one. With so many medications on the market and many being used off-label, there is the chance that not all medications received will work well. For those unfamiliar with the term off-label, this means a drug that was developed for a specific illness but was found to have beneficial effects for other illnesses. For example, one of the leading anti-inflammatory drugs on the market is Hydroxychloroquine or Plaquenil. This anti-malarial drug is found to be useful for connective tissue sufferers impacted by high levels of inflammation in their bodies. The drug slows the rate at which the inflammation rises and is helpful for most UCTD patients.

Inflammation in the body might present as swollen areas accompanied by pain and systemic fever or fever to the swollen area only. Prostaglandins[40] are responsible for

49

causing fever, pain and inflammation in the body. Consequently, medications are required to reduce the level of prostaglandins in the body thereby reducing or removing the offending inflammation. Commonly prescribed drugs include:

Non-Steroidal Anti-Inflammatory Disease Suppressants (NSAIDs)

Ibuprofen (Advil & Motrin), Naproxen (Aleve, Naprosyn & Midol Extended Relief), Diclofenac (Cataflam & Voltaren), Aspirin and COX-2 inhibitors (Celebrex) are just some of the NSAIDs available in the marketplace[41]. NSAIDs are useful for reducing inflammation as well as eliminating mild to moderate pain and fever in the patient. NSAID's are often available over the counter (OTC) and do not require prescriptions.

It is normally recommended that you take NSAIDs with food or prepare the stomach with proton pump inhibitors (Prilosec & Pevacid) [42] that reduce the levels of stomach acid. NSAIDs while useful can cause serious side effects in patients including bleeding stomachs, allergic reactions and kidney problems. Persons taking NSAIDs are also at risk for strokes and other cardiovascular issues.

Disease-Modifying Antirheumatic Drugs (DMARDs)

Hydroxychloroquine (Plaquenil), Methotrexate (MTX), Sulfasalazine and Leflonomide are all disease modifying drugs developed to slow the progression of the connective tissue disease[43]. Sulfasalazine and Plaquenil are first-line defense drugs typically prescribed to combat connective tissue issues. While not as strong as other DMARDs, Plaquenil as an anti-malarial drug has still been found useful in modifying and slowing the development of connective tissue diseases. Plaquenil is used when there is low disease activity and may be used for extended periods. However, due to concerns of the drug affecting eyes, regularly scheduled visits to the ophthalmologist is recommended

Stronger DMARDs like Leflonomide and MTX are known to be very effective and can be taken over long periods of time. MTX is taken once a week in oral or injectable form and should usually be taken in conjunction with folic acid to reduce the side effects. Common side effects include a feeling of malaise and dizziness. Unfortunately, although DMARDs like MTX are so effective with the disease management, they have serious side effects such as liver toxicity. DMARDs can cause birth defects should a woman become pregnant while on the drug. Usually a doctor has to make the decision if the benefits of taking the drugs outweigh the risks of the drug.

Biologics

Biological therapies (biologics) were developed from human genes to handle arthritic conditions that DMARDs were not able to help[44]. Biologics are immune suppressants. This class of drugs works faster than DMARDs and helps to prevent joint damage. Biologics are not oral pills as are most NSAIDs and DMARDs; rather, they are usually given in injection form. In some cases, biologics are given in tandem with MTX for maximum efficacy for the patient. Biologics are normally prescribed when the patient has high disease activity and has not been helped by other medications.

Common Biologics include Adalimumab (Humira), Etanercept (Enbrel), Abatacept (Orencia) and Infliximab (Remicade). While biologics have fewer side effects than DMARDS they do have the potential to cause more severe infections. Ensure that the doctor does liver tests before beginning you on a course of biologics as a means of establishing a baseline for future comparison.

Corticosteroids (Steroids)

Corticosteroids (steroids) mimic the naturally occurring human hormone cortisol [45]. Steroids are effective in reducing inflammation and by extension swelling and pain. Steroids suppress the immune system and are used to treat a variety of connective tissue diseases including lupus, Sjögren's RA and Scleroderma. Prednisone is one of the most commonly prescribed steroids and is given orally or by injection.

Prednisone like others in its class, are hydrocortisone based steroids. These steroids are synthetically produced to mimic hormones normally produced by the body's adrenals. Corticosteroids work by creating higher than normal levels of those hormones in the body thus suppressing inflammation.

Corticosteroids may be taken orally, by injection, topically or even nasally.

With UCTD, prednisone might be prescribed at low doses for medium to long-term use. In some cases, to treat a flare, your doctor might prescribe Methylprednisolone (Medrol pack) that works the same as prednisone but has anecdotally been reported to have lessened side effects than prednisone. During a flare, your doctor may also prescribe titrated higher doses of the steroids for 7-days or 14-days periods.

Please ensure that you follow the doctor's direction for weaning off steroids as improper weaning can lead to mild to severe withdrawal symptoms. While giving great benefit to CTD patients, steroids are known to cause side effects such as increased appetite and weight gain. Some patients report fat redistribution around their mid-section as a result of using steroids. Use of corticosteroids may result in central serous retinopathy (CSR) which causes serious eye impairment. Long-term steroid use can also lead to a 'moon face' or a rounded face over time.

My UCTD - My Medication History

Doctors will normally start you on Plaquenil and NSAIDs. Depending on how well you react to those medications or if your symptoms warrant it, doctors might introduce stronger drugs in the fight against the disease.

To date, I have taken Methotrexate, Prednisone, Plaquenil, Naproxen, Ibuprofen, Cataflam, Voltaren, Arcoxia, Mobic, Prednisone, Gabapentin and Celebrex among others. I have tried combinations, increased dosages, reduced dosages and I have still not found the magic combination to make me well. Some drugs like MTX have worked much better than others while others like Celebrex were a disaster.

At one point I was on both Plaquenil and Prednisone and I started to see men coming to get me. Do not laugh (but I know you are), but seriously, there were nights that I stood in the living room in the dark shaking like a leaf and hoping the men did not come and get me. Turns out I was having hallucinatory episodes caused by one or a combination of the medications. Once I came off the medications, my hallucinations disappeared. To this day I use this example in my lectures as an ice breaker. Imagine your lecturer telling you that she once saw men who did not exist, coming to get her? It makes for a fun ice breaker indeed.

Nasty side effects from some medications resulted in more symptoms and pain than before taking the medication. Case in point, after taking diclofenac oral tablets for year, I developed a sudden allergic reaction. Whether using the diclofenac topical cream or orally ingesting the tablet, I would break out in a rash and have the most severe gastrointestinal disturbances. Subsequently, I no longer take any medication with diclofenac such as Cataflam or Voltaren medications.

Over the years, I have developed several more allergies to different medications. When I first became ill and was prescribed medication, I didn't understand that I could call in and tell the doctor how I was reacting to the medication. I suffered much in those early years taking medication despite having what were some serious or at the least frightening side effects. After many bad experiences with some medications, I now report troublesome side effects to my doctor by at least the end of the first 2 weeks. It is therefore important to learn your body and your tolerances.

I had a situation where a doctor prescribed Methotrexate without warning me about the potential dangers of getting pregnant while on the drug. In another instance, I was prescribed medication containing diclofenac even though it was on my chart that I was allergic to the ingredient. Bactrim is another pill I was prescribed to handle my numerous infections. My reaction to the Bactrim was swift and severe as I went into an immediate flare. It turns out that John Hopkins Lupus Center also references the antibiotics Bactrim along with Septra as medications to avoid when you have Lupus or similar autoimmune conditions. Unfortunately one doctor did not take this advice into consideration when prescribing the Bactrim.

Bactrim caused me severe itching, muscle weakness & numbness and pain[46]. As such, I ensure I ask the doctor about the medication I am being prescribed instead of simply trusting that the doctor has all the answers. I am not advising you to ignore your doctor's advice, but I do ask that you consider that doctors are human and your health decisions are ultimately in your hand.

I do believe that some medications, Plaquenil and MTX among a select others, prove valuable if you can stick it out past the first 6 weeks. Incidentally, if I had judged MTX solely on how it made me feel in the initial 5 weeks (extreme nausea and vertigo) and stopped taking the drug, I would never have experienced the longest remission period I have had to date. Thus, if you can tolerate the side effects of a medication and most likely they will occur if only in mild form, you might find relief in the same medication your were willing to stop taking.

Take Charge of your Health

The key takeaway I want you to have after reading this chapter is that you must become involved in your health. I am not advocating hypochondriac behavior; however, you must be reasonably informed about the health options available to you.

The plethora of information on the Internet can be daunting. Some of the most prolific sites and blogs on autoimmune issues are run by non-medical persons. While I have discovered that these sites have useful information, I would not advise basing your health recovery plan solely on the anecdotal advice found on these sites. Do your research on reputable sites like the Mayo Clinic, WebMD, John Hopkins, The National Jewish Hospital and disease websites like scleroderma.org. If in doubt, stick to hospital websites, medical school sites, peer reviewed health publications or .gov health websites.

Document your symptoms and timeline of development so that it makes it easy for the doctor to delve into your health background. This also helps you avoid the fact that you are likely to forget some of the symptoms or issues while you are in the doctor's office. Bear in mind that not all doctors are appreciative of this tactic. I usually tell the doctor that with my memory issues, it is the best option for me to inform the doctor of all my issues thus providing the doctor with the full picture of my illness.

Additionally, I now document with pictures, my mysterious swellings and lumps, as these are not always visible at the time for my rheumy's appointment. Consider that your rheumy might have given you a six month visit schedule. Any symptom that arises during your wait for your next visit cannot be acknowledged unless it is a life or death situation or your rheumy decided to grant an emergency visit. Consequently, depending on the severity of the symptom, I either visit my local PCP or take pictures where possible for the rheumy to see on my next visit. I advise a similar plan to help your doctor better manage the symptoms that will invariable arise.

Let the doctor come to his or her own conclusion and do not try to tell the doctor what must be wrong with you. Trust me; this attitude never works well with doctors. Have a reasonable discussion with the doctor where possible but never try to tell the doctor his or her job. It would be better to find another doctor if you feel the doctor is wrong or not listening to you.

Do not feel that you must take every medication suggestion from a doctor. Again, have a frank discussion with the doctor if you are uncomfortable with the thought of taking a certain medication. I have refused medication based on cost and potential side effects and my doctor was able to prescribe alternatives. In some cases, where I am unsure about a medicine I ask my pharmacist about potential issues the doctor might have forgotten to tell me.

I must caution you not to spend too much time on the Internet reading up on your medications. I find that some knowledge is good but the pursuit of too much information on your medications can have negative effects on your health journey. I know persons who spend time checking every side effect of the medications they are prescribed. While it is good to know which medication you are prescribed, I find that some persons suffer from every side effect that they read about.

Your mind is a powerful thing and it is possible to manifest reactions to medications due to constant worry and fretfulness over the medicine. Please understand that this why some doctors are skeptical when patients tell them the entire list of side effects and then proceed to claim each one of the side effects as happening to them. In no way am I rubbishing the fact that there might be a genuine side effect. However, I must ensure you understand that sometimes it is possible to self-sabotage.

« CHAPTER 4: FAMILY & FRIENDS »

Let me preface this section by saying I have gotten great support from close friends and family members around me. However, I have had more naysayers, negative and toxic persons in my life that all decided that they knew more than the doctors. The less that people understand about connective tissue disease, the greater their level of antipathy towards your illness.

I must caution newly diagnosed persons with UCTD and other connective tissue disease to manage their expectations of support from your circle of friends and family. If I have learnt nothing else, I have learnt to quickly weed out of my circle, any person who through idle words or actions, try to become my doctor or psychiatrist (and no I do not see a psychiatrist).

This disease is not easy to understand. After a decade of suffering with this disease, despite well over 60 doctor visits, despite trying well over 30 different types of medications (trying does not mean being a medication junkie), I still do not fully understand UCTD as it is ever changing.

The changing nature of the disease makes it difficult for people to comprehend the changes happening in your body. I find that it makes some persons suspicious as to whether or not you are attempting to garner attention. For me, getting up one morning and seeing only blurred outlines was simply another symptom I seemed to have manufactured. I believe some persons were genuinely surprised to see me in glasses as that meant I actually might have been telling the truth.

I have reached a point in my journey that even as an adult, I carry my mother or husband along to doctor visits so that they too can hear what the doctors tell me. This is not because these two wonderful persons disbelieve me, but rather, it does provide me with an additional layer of "protection" against those who believe I am paraphrasing or lying about what the doctor said.

On January 1st 2007, a family friend called me to wish me Happy New Year and ask if I wasn't planning to stop playing sick and go back to work. At that time, my joints hurt so badly that I couldn't bend them and my fatigue levels were so high that I could not even maintain a proper conversation for any extended stretch of time.

I hate being sick. My Type A personality has a lot to get accomplished and it does hurt at times to see the callousness displayed by some persons. Nonetheless, I remind myself that some of these persons mean well but lack knowledge, some simply lack empathy and some are just plain mean.

The majority of persons around you will have no clue how to handle your illness. It is quite likely that you will find yourself missing events and this is one of the biggest complaints I think friends and families have against persons who suffer from UCTD and other connective tissue diseases. How do you tell them that being in the sun might make you more ill?

How do you get them to understand that too much activity takes a toll on the body in ways they cannot understand or may never experience?

Nothing however, quite annoyed me like someone telling me that I was behaving sick like I had cancer. At no point have I wished for, nor acted as if I had cancer. My suffering is real to me even though my diagnosis is not cancer. I am unsure when cancer became the yardstick by which other illnesses are measured. I applaud cancer survivors and I see the real life and death struggle they face. Notwithstanding, I refuse to cower or hide or be silenced about discussing and finding a cure for connective tissue diseases, specifically UCTD.

Our illness is probably one of the least understood connective tissue diseases, but we are real people suffering in real ways. I no longer accommodate any one telling me how I should feel. Do not let people dictate your feelings to you. The feelings are yours, take control of your feelings and despite your challenges, daily remind yourself of your worth. After all, our challenges do make us stronger.

Dealing with Inconsiderate Statements

There is a reason I hate going to funerals and repasts- I never know the correct words to say. In the same vein, consider that some persons do not know the correct things to say to you. Of course some persons speak without thinking, while others do mean to be cutting and belittling. My pet peeves are in order of annoyance:

But you don't look sick

Persons with chronic illnesses often experience this statement, which while seemingly easy to ignore, can be become irritating and downright annoying over time. I wonder if persons telling me I don't look sick ever considered that they do not see me when I am really sick and writhing in pain- that is what the doctor is for. I stay home and indoors when I am ill and so I suppose it makes it harder to convince persons that I am ill when they never see me when I am in tears or my joints are swollen.

I heard you were sick but you do not look sick is a statement I have grown to detest. Do I have to look emaciated, haggard, pasty or walking with a stick to be taken seriously? Believe me, I have heard it all. "How is it you are sick and haven't lost weight?" You see, losing weight means you are sick; at least in Jamaica it does. Persons asking these questions never seem to consider that medications can cause the UCTD patient to actually gain weight. My suggestion, take a minute to explain to them how illnesses and medication can contribute to weight gain.

I have always considered the statement, "but your face doesn't look sick" as another asinine statement. I mean, how exactly should a sick face look? Fortunately for persons making such statement, I have realized that they simply do not grasp the concept of an invisible chronic illness. They do not understand that there are periods of great days and other bleak periods that are the bane of our existence. As such, I now practice sharing knowledge about the illness. I am now able to give them an elevator speech about how chronic illnesses are not always as apparent by examining one's face and how a supportive attitude helps the chronic sufferer. Remember an elevator speech is concise but includes all the major elements of the message. After all, you do not want to bore or overwhelm friends and family, but you do need to inform them so they are better able to be supportive.

The Spoon Theory mentioned later in this chapter deals with how to explain to friends and family about your health challenges and this hopefully will be beneficial for you to add in your own version of your elevator speech.

Well, it could be worse/ Chin up, it isn't so bad/It's not like you have lupus

I call UCTD the 'not' disease. You will hear many times that at least you do 'not' have cancer, lupus, RA et cetera (you fill in the blanks). In an almost dismissive way, persons will tell you that you have no real worries as your disease is 'not' that serious. I am actually grateful that UCTD is 'not' that serious and life threatening but that does not remove the multiple symptoms- the mild to severe pain, the inflammation, the swellings and the muscle weakness that we UCTD patients experience on a daily basis.

Just get some fresh air and you will be fine/ if you exercise you will feel better

Seriously, you really think fresh air is the cure all? Or better yet, that exercise will make me better in no time? Think again, it is not that simple. I have had periods where I walked anything between 1-3 miles daily with no issues while another week, 15 minutes of walking brings me pain, lightheadedness and fatigue. I think my issues are compounded because I have both UCTD and FMS and FMS is known as possibly causing exercise intolerance[47]. This simply means I sometimes feel much worse after exercising than better even though conventional wisdom says I should feel fine.

 In order to stay fit, my rheumy had cleared me for low impact exercises[48] such swimming and gentle walking but it seems to some persons I wasn't doing enough. "Come on," they said, "you need to run or do some aerobics in order to get your body moving." Stupidly, I discarded my doctor's advice and joined the gym. In short order instead of feeling better, I was doing worse. Cardio was fun but my body rebelled, I got dizzy with cold sweats and chills as I followed the recommended cardio routine.

Meanwhile in the weight room, I explained my joint issues and a past broken shoulder to the certified trainer, but I was assured I just had to build muscle and strength and it would result in me feeling so much better. A scant 6 weeks later, I was worse than when I joined the gym. I had swollen joints and extreme fatigue as it turned out, my body couldn't handle the stress of the gym. Lesson learnt, let others do what they must while I listen to my body and I advise you to do the same.

Go vegan/vegetarian and you will feel better

Where do I begin? Could it be as simple as removing animal protein from my diet? I had tried years ago with no success, so summer 2012 was the time for a new try. Well, apart from missing my meat and dreaming about it, I saw no noticeable difference over a 3 month period of abstaining from meat and gluten. Some say I should have gone longer, but as I read for myself, after the first 6-8 weeks, I should have started seeing some benefit in symptoms, however minute.

I do however eat less meat and I have incorporated more nuts, legumes and non-meat options in my diet as I believe in moderation and a balanced diet. There are numerous books and sites that offer anecdotal stories on how vegan or raw foods can cure autoimmune issues. I have nothing against persons who abstain from eating meat, but I refuse to be vilified because I chose to.

I have no doubt that eating more wholesome plant-based foods will make you healthier. Eating more whole non-processed foods and organic fruits, vegetables and meats will contribute to our general health. However, I have seen no clinical studies offering proof that a vegan/vegetarian lifestyle will cure you of UCTD.

More so, I know vegans and vegetarians who for years practiced the lifestyle yet became ill nonetheless and manifested symptoms of cancer and lifestyle diseases among others. As such, I reiterate that there is no one "right" way for everyone. Our bodies make the choices; it is not always up to us and our diet.

Of course, a plant-based lifestyle might remove the triggers for some sufferers; thus "curing" them. However, with UCTD, no single cure exists. Consequently, the risk factors for autoimmune conditions are far to varied to center on food choices as being the only way to find a cure. If anyone tries to tell you otherwise, then there is a bridge being sold for pennies somewhere and I would like to buy it.

You just need to eat garlic/ build your immune system

The dumbest thing I did when I first got ill was to listen to persons around me and herbal practitioners who convinced me to take more immune building supplements. FAIL! According to the John Hopkins Lupus Centre, building the immune system is the last thing CTD patients should be doing if they want to be well[45]. I now know part of the reason why I was getting worse and not better all those years. It turns out that like other CTD patients, I have an overactive immune system that needs to be suppressed not heightened.

Garlic is just one of those great immune boosters that are beneficial to healthy persons, not so much so to most UCTD sufferers. Months of taking Echinacea and garlic did not actually improve my health as I was only putting my already overactive immune system into overdrive. One other commonly recommended immune booster is the over the counter supplement melatonin (to promote sleep). Melatonin did not give me the desired result and actually was interacting with my medications and might have contributed to my hormonal issues at the time.

Accordingly, I can only caution against listening to persons doling out health advice unless you have researched the advice yourself or cleared it with your doctor.

You are not taking enough vitamins/taking the right vitamins

On the issue of taking more vitamins, some persons take so many vitamins that it is almost like they are eating another meal. I have seen persons taking 20+ vitamins and supplements twice a day and unsurprising to me, it doesn't always guarantee good health. I believe in taking vitamins but I refuse to become a vitamin junkie.

Vitamins are great additions to your diet but which vitamins and the amount that you should consume in unclear to me. Furthermore the vitamin industry is largely unregulated and so all vitamins are not made the same. Which ones to take and on what basis? This is still something I am still trying to figure out.

Vitamin D levels are suspected to be low in UCTD patients. Some doctors recommend taking 10,000 units of Vitamin D daily to see optimal benefits[49]. However, at the urgings of some non-traditional health practitioners and acquaintances, I have been told that I need to take in excess of 40,000 units a day in order to be well. Bear in mind that this amount far exceeds daily recommended rates for Vitamin D which is known to have side effects at too high a dosage[50]. Possible side effects of high levels of Vitamin D include calcification of tissue and the vascular system and can lead to heart arrhythmias. Again, I caution the reader to do his or her own research before a wholesale acceptance of what you have been told anecdotally.

The Spoon Theory - Explaining to Friends & Family

This disease baffles doctors and scientists. With all the reading you have done you remain confused about UCTD. Can you honestly then, expect your friends and families to easily understand this disease? I find the best introduction to explaining UCTD to your circle is by having them read The Spoon Theory written by Christine Miserandino[51].

In this article, Christine chronicles her struggles and how something as simple as spoons were helpful in her explaining to her best friend how this illness robs her of her energy and options. The article is a good read and one recommended for all chronic illness sufferers.

The premise behind the spoon theory is that we as autoimmune sufferers have a limited amount of spoons; each spoon representing a part of our life. Conversely, healthy persons have endless spoons; allowing them more possibilities. As autoimmune sufferers, we are normally out of spoons before being able to complete the day's tasks. This is often difficult for us to accept.

Imagine then, how difficult it is for our families to understand and accept our illness. Thus, one of the most pressing issues I face is relating the illness in a way that family and friends understand. I like the Spoon Theory as it eloquently states in layman's terms, the difficulties and challenges persons with chronic illnesses face.

Someone once told me the Spoon Theory did not apply to my condition as the author of the theory was referencing lupus. In reality, the Spoon Theory highlights the same struggles that UCTD patients' experience. I explain UCTD as having to plan a full 12-hour day with only 6 hours available to get the same tasks done.

In my scenario, the UCTD sufferer sees the full slate of daily activities ahead but is unable to complete all the tasks due to possible pain, swelling and fatigue. Instead, the UCTD sufferer must now prioritize which activities are attainable within the reduced hours.

My personal experience is that on my business website Buy Jamaica Stores, I sell Jamaican items and ship globally. Some days whilst on business errands, I would find myself napping or resting in the car while parked at one of my suppliers. I cannot tell you how many times I had received strange looks for doing so. It wasn't that I wanted to lay there with insufficient energy to complete my tasks. That would be far from accurate.

I often leave home with high energy levels. After a 30-minute drive and two stops at my suppliers, my energy levels either dips suddenly or I experience a gradual decline in my energy levels. Either way, on numerous occasions, I have had to repurpose my day. As a UCTD sufferer you know 'that today's unresolved tasks must still be accomplished and so tomorrow's schedule has additional work to be added. If you could not manage the work today, is it even possible to handle it tomorrow?

It is usually at this juncture that healthy persons tell you to just push through. In some cases, persons with other illnesses or even persons that share your illness will also tell you that if they can do it then you can do it too. Believe me, I am a firm believer in pushing through pain. I have reached for lofty goals even when hurting. Despite this, I can unequivocally state that a sure way for my body to "crash" is to push through some days.

Consider that your body may differ from mine and the severity of our illnesses may also differ. For me, my perception of pain is heightened due to my FMS diagnosis, so even though my brain recognizes that the pain should not be as bad, try sending that memo to my body.

Your body's propensity to handle stressors is not determined by what others think. Gently explain to your friends and family members that you do have limitations. Establish gentle boundaries and be willing to explain in a loving way how your illness has redefined you.

Some persons will note that the illness does not define them, to the point that it is almost a mantra. I disagree, my illness has redefined me. It has redefined my boundaries and limitations. While I am not my illness, my new persona has learnt to embrace my illness even while embracing a new outlook.

The Impact on Family Members & Close Friends

How many times have your seen your family members or friends cry because of your illness? Have you noticed the stress caused when your family and friends cannot help you get well? Recognize that your illness does not only affect you.

As part of a family unit, your pain and discomfort will sometimes affect family members. Family members and friends, have a vested interest in seeing you well. Therefore accord your family members and friends some slack when they err in how they respond to your illness.

Often times, family members and friends are overwhelmed. They see that you are ill but cannot comprehend the circumstances around the illness. Just as we grieve because we have this disease, so do some family and friends. Allow them to grieve for what they think they have lost. It may be that they think they have lost an ally, a friend, that sister who would always come shopping, or the husband who would take pleasure in cutting the yard.

Understand that the limitations you feel have now been transferred to your family. It might be hard for your familial unit to see the once vivacious and outgoing personality dimmed. Unfortunately to some, your limitations might be viewed as depression or laziness. Try to help them see that that characterization is faulty; gently show them why you are unable to function as before.

Some of the changes in the family might be financial. This disease takes a serious financial toll on many of us. The cost of medications and seeing the doctors, the innumerable tests and the lost wages can affect even the most stable relationships. For a person used to earning a salary to being dependent on disability, the change can be devastating.

How does the decision to take disability benefits affect your household? What money earning venture can you conceive that is still within your current abilities? Have a frank discussion on finances with your partner and children and extended family members where needed. After all, your bills might become their bills and they all must have a say into how the family income is spent.

I am going to be blunt and say that this illness sometimes makes some UCTD sufferers into victims. Such persons adopt a victim mentality and a woe-is-me mindset. This mindset is not conducive in helping to mitigate the blow that this disease will cause the family.

While your family and friends might love you, they are not beholden to you. I have seen situations where marriages fail because the sick partner makes everything about him or her. I believe that no matter how sick we each become, we should always consider the other persons in our relationships. Once we start thinking about other persons than ourselves, we can better see through their eyes.

« CHAPTER 5: MANAGING UCTD »

UCTD might be a permanent part of our lives. As such, we have to learn how best to manage the disease. Having this disease does not mean that we should allow the disease to control us; instead, we must develop the ability to manage the disease.

Exercise - Get Moving & Stay Moving

Change your activities to reduce stress on your body and joints. Do not sit at your desk too long as that may result in exacerbating UCTD issues like circulation and encourage swelling of the ankles. Involve yourself in low impact exercises such as walking and swimming. Keeping active is essential when you have UCTD or any connective tissue disease. In most cases, milder exercises might be more beneficial to you. Some persons are able to master more involved exercises and compete in marathons but it is essentially up to you how you manage your body.

Exercise does not have to be difficult nor does it have to be for extended periods of time. While 30 minutes of activity is recommended for optimal health, understand and listen to your body. If you can only manage 15 minutes, then those 15 minutes of activity is better than none. Where it is not possible to go outside, then invest into a game system like the

Wii that along with the balance board and the right exercise DVD, allows you to customize a workout suitable to your condition.

I can caution against trying to do intensive boot camp type workouts without consulting your doctor. I know healthy persons who tore ligaments and sprained ankles trying to keep up with these high intensity workouts. UCTD affects persons differently so there will always be those UCTD sufferers who are able to engage in certain exercises that you cannot. Pace yourself and listen to your body. Check your local community center or YMCA for activity classes. Do not be embarrassed to join the senior citizen's exercise programs; trust me, they still can probably outdo you.

I once created an intensive Wii Active exercise program that included 20 minutes of simulated tennis. I managed perfectly well for the first two days but day three saw me in bed with swollen shoulders and intense pain. Similar results happened whenever I changed from milder exercises to more involved intensive and repetitive exercises. Consequently, I learnt my lesson. I now keep it simple and no more than 30 to 45 minutes of walking at least 5 days a week.

Dealing with Pain

Chronic Pain is pain that lasts longer than three months. UCTD patients usually suffer from chronic pain, namely headaches and joint pains. A UCTD diagnosis means that you will be dealing with chronic pain for as long as you have the disease. One of the easiest ways persons deal with chronic pain is by taking medication. The pharmaceutical industry is aware that a growing number of persons suffer from chronic pain. In response, the pharmaceutical industry developed pain pills to help sufferers deal with this pain.

What however, if there were other ways to handle your chronic pain? Would you be interested to learn? Would you be willing to give up your pain pills and what for some has become a dependency? Over the years, I have discovered and tried techniques that have helped me better manage my pain and reduce the need for daily pain pills. These five techniques are given below:

Change Your Attitude

My childhood friend Jessica B. taught me the concept of smile and nod. As children, I was always more hot tempered than she was and was always ready to do battle and defend the underdog. Even as we grew older, she would take a softer, gentler approach to life while I employed my normal, no-holds barred temperament. I am a straight shooter- I say it and I mean it.

One thing I took away from my friendship with Jessie was that she would always try to calm me by saying smile and nod. At first, I thought it the most ridiculous thing I had heard. Why smile and let things slide when you can simply set the record straight or deal with it head-on? I confess it took me years to get the underlying concept.

When you smile and nod, you are in essence, adopting a more Zen-like attitude and creating a more relaxed sense of being. This concept however, does not mean you have to physically smile and nod, nor does it mean you have to be acquiescent with everything. Remember, the energy it takes to be combative is not always worth it.

As a chronic pain sufferer, you will need to learn to entertain a positive outlook and think positive thoughts. This positivity actually helps to put you in a better frame of mind to deal with your pain. Additionally, negative emotions and stress can exacerbate your pain. Consequently, it is advisable to smile and nod when petty situations would otherwise aggravate you.

Find a Support Group

Misery likes company they say. If that is so, chronic pain sufferers should be happy together. One of the best things I did was to find and join support groups. There were no UCTD support groups that I was aware of in Jamaica. As a result, I found online support groups that I thought could provide me with both support and information.

During the initial phases of my illness when I didn't know what was wrong with me, I didn't know which group was the best to join. I felt like a fraud joining a lupus group as I didn't have a lupus diagnosis. I left that group and then joined a RA group but found members were more interested in seeing who was taking the most pills. I couldn't understand why it was a competition to see who had the most ailments.

I was happy later on to find great support groups on Daily Strength and Inspire. Even though I later left these groups for a more intimate and dedicated UCTD on Facebook, I found great support on both those sites. The benefits of a support group are:

1.   **Similar persons** - do you know how great it feels when you talk about a symptom that your doctor had rubbished and someone in the forum understands? Sometimes another member has similar symptoms and can even give you the medical name for it. In one case, I was better equipped for my next doctor's appointment as I could give the doctor a clue as to what he should be testing for.

2.   **It is cathartic** – you are able to rant among persons who share your frustration and pain (literally). It is a "safe" area where you will not be judged. You can vent, cry and "anonymously" express yourself without fear of involving friends and family members. In my FB support group, persons can write in the group without sharing with their wider FB list thus keeping their private health business separate from their FB profile.

3.   **Discuss what works for others** – let me begin with a caution, do NOT take medical advice from non-medical persons. There is nothing wrong with discussing your medication routine and hearing suggestions, however do not adjust your medication based on a stranger's advice. I can understand if the discussion is about supplements or other

non-prescription products, as I began taking turmeric based on a recommendation from a group member. Even with the recommendation, I made sure to do my own research before taking the supplement.

There is a wealth of knowledge in the support forum. Learn about alternative therapies that others have tried, discuss anti-inflammatory diets and get tips on how others manage this illness. My recommendation is to find a support group that works for you. I am told some support groups have bullies and if that is so, leave those groups. You are not beholden to join and remain in any group in which you are uncomfortable. There are plenty other groups online. Remember you are in a group to find a certain degree of healing.

Understand your Pain

How bad is your pain on a daily basis? Could you assign a number to your pain? If you are wondering why on earth I am asking you about assigning a number to your pain, let me explain. Even though you suffer from chronic pain, your pain levels may vary daily. You will discover it is easier to mentally manage your pain if you learn to categorize your pain using a pain scale.

If you have ever been evaluated at work using a rating scale, then the concept of a pain scale should be familiar to you. The pain scale is numbered 1 to 10 with 10 being the worst pain you have ever had in your life (childbirth, bad toothache, surgery etc.). There is a popular facial representation pictorial relating your facial expression to your pain levels. You may visit Wong-Baker Faces Foundation for more information[52]. Personally, I use a simple rating scale to judge my pain levels:

0 to 2 (mild pain)

I take no pills for mild pain. I use my pain management techniques and distract myself.

3 to 5 (moderate pain)

I take pills only if I am doing very involved mental work. Otherwise, I use imagery or music to help me cope.

6 to 8 (moderate to severe pain)

Sometimes, I take one of my milder prescription pills. It depends on whether my other methods of blocking or managing pain are successful or not. Mild pain pills are usually helpful with pain level 6. By the time my pain reaches pain level 8; I need either stronger pain pills or combine a non-medical therapy with a milder pain pill.

9 to 10 (severe pain)

At this pain level, I cannot concentrate, I get very nauseous and body is coated with a light sheen of perspiration. I have to take my strongest pain pills and at times, I also have to add topical creams or a cold/hot compress therapy. Sleep, if possible, helps tremendously.

Once you can establish your 10, then rationalize your pain in relation to the 10 (the worst pain). It makes your pain more manageable if you realize that pain level 5 is actually a good day for you (when rationalized against pain level 8 days). It is a good idea to maintain a journal to record your daily pain levels (or you could use a spreadsheet). This journal can provide insight into your daily pain levels and help the doctor decide the best pain medication management program for you.

Using the pain scale, I usually only take a pain pill when I perceive a pain in the moderate to severe category. The pain scale helps me keep in the severity of my pain in context, and thus I am better able to judge what tasks I can still complete. There are days when I tell myself that my pain is simply not bad enough and that is sufficient for my brain to help redirect my attention to tasks instead of the pain. However, on really bad days, no amount of 'talking" with my brain is enough to mask or ignore the pain.

When I visit my doctor, the discussion of pain sometimes centers on the type of pain. Once I have identified my pain level, I still need to explain how the pain feels. Pain varies and could range from a dull pain to throbbing pain[53]. What are the different types of pain that you experience? Could you explain how your pain differs? Why not familiarize yourself with the types and classifications for the variations in your pain.

Chronic Pain – long-term pain that can range from mild to severe; may also be daily pain.

Dull Ache – a distant feeling mild ache that can normally be overlooked.

Throbbing Pain – a pain that changes in intensity; may pound or seemingly beat to a rhythm. This type of pain is normally mild to severe pain that spikes in intensity at intervals.

Sharp Pain – severe pain that causes extreme discomfort. This discomfiting pain may be so excruciating that it is both physically and mentally distressing.

Steady Pain – this pain may be more of a mild to moderate pain that remains unchanged in its intensity.

Breakthrough Pain – a more severe pain that occurs even though the chronic pain sufferer is taking pain medications. In other words, the pain breaks through the expected medication relief period.

Burning Pain – this pain normally occurs in tandem with the peripheral neuropathy issues that some autoimmune sufferers experience. This pain feels like a combination between pain and a burning sensation. The pain is often more uncomfortable than it is severe.

Once you have identified your pain type, it is still useful to understand the underlying reason behind the pain. Your pain is not simply chronic pain. Rather, your pain is caused by:

Tissue damage & inflammation – known as nociceptive pain, this pain occurs due to the physical or perceived damage to the body's tissues. As inflammation levels rise in the body, so too might the patient's pain levels. Nociceptive pain can range from a dull pain to throbbing pain and may be worsened by movement of the affected area.

Nerve damage – with autoimmune conditions, some patients do have neuropathic symptoms. Neuropathic pain causes a burning pain that is accompanied by a feeling of pins and needles or numbness in the affected area. This type of pain normally happens as a result of damaged nerves and anomalous nerve signals being sent to part of the body.

Psychologically-driven factors – some pain is psychogenic in nature. This pain occurs when stress on the body results in pain or the brain "remembers" pain that once occurred. As discussed later in the chapter, the body will sometimes become used to the pain. Consequently, even in the absence of real pain, the body reacts as if it still hurts.

With all the discussion of pain and pains scales, please remember that everyone feels or perceives pain differently. Some persons are stoic in relation to pain and have what might be termed a high pain threshold. Our pain threshold might be primarily biological but our psyche plays an important role in how we perceive pain. The bodies of persons with chronic pain have learnt to feel pain; the body becomes hypersensitized.

According to Whitten, Donovan and Cristobal (2005), "Patients with chronic pain have reduced pain thresholds and therefore feel pain more intensely."[54] Consequently, never get into a debate with someone about how your pain feels. You may however try our next tip on handling pain in order to rewire how you think about pain.

Biofeedback

As the body becomes hypersensitized to pain, it becomes necessary to retrain the body to deal with pain. Biofeedback is non-invasive and involves wearing sensors that provide your brain with information about your bodily function. Using these sensors, you can learn to recognize what is happening in the body and in time learn to control your body functions. This rewiring occurs as over time, the body learns to behave differently and acts in line with what the brain trained it to do. According to the Mayo clinic, biofeedback uses the mind to improve the health of the body[55]. Personally, I have not tried this technique yet, but I am adding it to my list of techniques to try in the coming year.

Guided Imagery & Distractions

Have you ever imagined yourself on a beach somewhere? Did your imagination get so detailed that you could almost hear the waves lap the shores and smell the ocean? Or have you ever imagined eating a slice of cake and it became so real that you could almost taste the cake?

If you have done anything like I mentioned above, you already have the basis to begin guided imagery. Guided imagery is focusing the mind and relaxing the body. By taking deep breaths and picturing a special scene in your thoughts, you are able to have your mind drift away despite the pain you might be feeling. Spend 10 to 15 minutes engaging your mind peacefully and see if your see a difference.

During your session, ask yourself questions that will evoke details. How does the place look, smell or feel? Are there people there? As you use the answers to the question to build your peaceful place, let yourself visit for a while. Once you are finished, try to carry those peaceful feelings back to the present with you. For those who find it difficult to do on your own, you may seek out audio materials to help you.

Distraction is similar to the guided imagery as you must distract yourself from the pain. Common distractions may include involving yourself in a detailed task, playing a game, getting immersed in a book or a movie, listen to music or immersing yourself in social media activities. The premise is that the brain can only handle a limited amount of stimuli and thus distractions pull the brain's awareness away from the pain.

Alternative Therapies

Body Massages, Lymphatic Drainage & Reflexology

Massages are useful for relaxation and healing. With various forms of massages, it is up to the patient to choose the most suitable massage for the condition. It is thought that massages help to reduce endorphins that help chronic pain sufferers manage pain and reduce use of pain pills. Massages are also thought to help relieve stress in the body and promote a better mood. In this section, I will speak to deep tissue and Swedish massages as two of the massage options available to you.

Deep tissue massages use deep and slow kneading of the deep muscle layers. Sometimes the muscles and connected tissue are knotted. The only way to release the tension is by having a deep tissue massage. The massage therapist will use the palm as well as the elbow, the forearm or the knuckles. Sometimes the deep muscles and tendons are so tightly knotted that they can impede circulation and cause pain. Deep tissue massage gives the correct pressure needed to reach these knotted bands of muscle and connective tissue.

In contrast, a Swedish massage uses gentle superficial kneading motions of the hand of the masseuse can help to relax the muscle and the body. This form of massage also includes gentle movement of the joints to improve movement. I confess that I have fallen asleep on numerous occasions while getting one of these massages. Swedish massages are excellent de-stressors after a trying week

Reflexology can be loosely considered as a form of massage. Reflexology involves massaging the soles of the feet, the palms of the hand and in some cases the ears of the patient. Reflexology is based on the premise that entire body is connected and that the joints and organs of the body can be "massaged" by using reflexology.

Each section of the sole of the feet, the palms and the ears corresponds with a part of the body. Reflexologists therefore use an established pictorial chart that explains which parts correspond to the respective joint or organ. For example, the tops of the toes correspond with the sinuses. The idea is that by applying specific pressure in that spot, the patient's sinuses should be positively affected.

My Alternative Therapy Journey

I have been having reflexology sessions since 2007 and while it hasn't healed me as I hoped, I have seen benefits from my sessions. To be fair, I combine a lymphatic drainage massage along with the reflexology in a hour and a half session. Here in Jamaica, my reflexologist, Mrs. Shirley Reeson was the first to suggest an autoimmune issue. Each time I went for a session, she would feel what she termed nodules under my skin or what felt like rice grains on the soles of my feet. She deduced that I was having an autoimmune reaction and suggested I mention it to my doctor.

Unfortunately for me, mentioning to the doctor that I thought I had an autoimmune issues based on the word of an alternative medicine practitioner did not bode well for me. Two different doctors thought I was being a hypochondriac. After all, how dare my reflexologist try to diagnose me? By now you might have surmised that Shirley was correct and those Kooks were wrong.

Shirley 1- Doctors 0

In another instance, more than two years before my vision issues, Shirley again suggested that the pain I was experiencing at a certain spot on my soles meant I should have my eyes checked. I went to the ophthalmologist and everything seemed normal. I did not yet know that this visit become very important. A year later when my vision changed, my ophthalmologist was able to use the report from my earlier visit as a baseline of how badly and how quickly my eyesight had changed. Thanks again Shirley.

Shirley 2- Doctors 0

In conjunction with the reflexology, lymphatic drainage has helped me as I would sometimes get very painful lymph nodes and terrible pains around the breast. I found that even though the lymphatic drainage did not halt my joint pains, I got relief from swollen and painful lymph nodes within 24 hours after the session. I must confess that the hours immediately following the session were brutal. My body felt like I had completed vigorous exercise. However, as with the concept of "after the storm comes the calm", so did my body react- I felt better in a few hours.

Initially, when I started having joint pains, I was prompted to start getting regular massages for what some saw as me being stressed thus being in pain. I tried a few massage sessions and quickly discovered that regular Swedish massages were nice but they were not the healing massages I needed. I then tried the deep tissue massage and discovered, NEVER do a deep tissue massage when you are in pain. I felt like a truck had run over my body and I did not see any improvements. A deep tissue massage is even more painful and harmful if you have an overlapping fibromyalgia diagnosis. Some persons disagree with this view but I can attest to feeling worse after a deep tissue massage and hurting for days.

If you need to find a massage practitioner, I recommend doing a Google search and read reviews on the potential massage place or on the therapist. Reviews are an excellent way to determine if you will get good service. While in the USA, I used Google to find a licensed practitioner near my location. Be advised that a person licensed to do massages may not be certified to do lymphatic drainage or reflexology.

Acupuncture

According to the Britain's NHS website, "Acupuncture is a form of ancient Chinese medicine in which fine needles are inserted into the skin at certain points on the body" (2012, ¶1)[56]. Acupuncture is a centuries-old practice where practitioners try to unblock the body's meridians and enable the Qi (pronounced chi or chee) to flow freely around the body. The Qi is considered the essential life force in the body and any blockage of the Qi is thought to result in illness.

Ensure you visit a licensed acupuncturist and do not feel afraid as there should be no pain when done correctly. Currently based on scientific evidence, acupuncture is only recommended for lower back pain. Anecdotally however, acupuncture is said to remedy migraines, fertility issues, joint pains and swellings

I have friends that swear by acupuncture and to be honest I have not given it a try in the last 5 years. However in the early days of my illness, I did regular sessions. For the most part I had no issues with the needles, it didn't hurt. However, any needle near my gluteal areas (buttocks) would feel like someone had hammered a large nail. After multiple tries and multiple sessions, I finally called halt to acupuncture session. Every other part of my body was fine except for that one area that would not allow the acupuncturist to place any needles there. My orthopedic and rheumatic doctors would both later tell me that the area was a known fibromyalgia tender point.

Home Remedies & Supplements

In the absence of medication, there are several home remedies and supplements that may be used to reduce pain and inflammation.

Applying hot and cold compresses alternately to swollen and painful joints can help tremendously. Begin with cold and alternate with the hot ensuring that you leave the compress on for about 30-40 seconds each. Be cautious in handling the hot compress and take care in applying to the skin. Do not put too hot a compress on the skin.

Old school compress methods require a basin with cold water and ice and a basin with hot water. Using two different small towels wet the towels in each basin respectively and apply as directed. If the hot compress is too hot, then place the wet compress in a larger towel to reduce the heat before placing directly on the skin.

Wintergreen alcohol and Epsom salt combined to create a mixture that is good for applying to swollen and painful joints. You can purchase premade solutions from your pharmacy such as CVS or online at Amazon. Alternatively, you can make your own by combining half bottle of wintergreen with 1 ½ cups of Epson salt. Shake the mixture well before each use.

Use natural plants and herbs such as Aloe Vera and in tropical and sub-tropical climates we have a plant we call leaf of life (Tree of Life, Life Leaf, Air Plant, Miracle Leaf, Aporo, Kalanchoe); both plants being useful in reducing joint swelling. Using the natural Aloe Vera, peel the skin and create a mush out of the pulp. Apply to the skin and bandage securely but not too tightly. Repeat twice a day as needed. The leaf of life leaf or juice may be used. If using the leaf, gently heat over a flame (candle is best) before applying to the inflamed joint.

Both the leaf of life and Aloe Vera grow in my backyard and so I am fortunate to be able to have access to these plants. I am told that pure Aloe Vera Gel works in a similar manner to the pure plant, but I have not tried it myself.

Consider supplements such as Turmeric, Krill Oil, Devils Claw, and Cat's Claw among others. If you are considering anything outside of your vitamin supply, contemplate adding anti-inflammatory supplements to your regimen. Anti-inflammatory supplements are just one more way to help your body heal more naturally. Some persons forgo conventional medicines to take supplements but I cannot guide you down that path.

During Easter 2013, after a bad reaction to a combination of medicines - Plaquenil, Cymbalta for my Fibro, Meloxicam and Prednisone, I gave up on pills. I was frustrated. In response I asked my doctor to take me off the pills and I decided to only use alternative therapy and disease management techniques. Despite taking Turmeric twice daily, adding two to four Krill oil pills daily, adding Devil's claw, a probiotic, a prenatal and Vitamin D 2000 units per day, I still kept getting sicker. Unfortunately this time around, I have had to add MTX as unconventional techniques alone were not helping.

I hope my experience serves to show that not everything that works for one person will work the same way for another. As such, do not get disappointed when the "recommended' herbal alternatives do not give you the breakthrough you desired. Although I did not get the breakthrough I wanted while on supplements, I still take them as I believe I see an improvement when I take them over the periods in which I did not. Keep trying, try new recommended supplements, adjust supplement dosages and above all, keep your doctor informed of your supplement list.

I seriously do advise boosting your anti-inflammatory fight with select supplements. Be careful and investigate ingredients prior to using supplements in the event that you have an allergy to a particular supplement or the supplement interacts with your medication. Choose supplements from established companies and read the ingredient list to ensure there are no fillers that might cause allergies to you. Some supplements might have in trace amounts of gluten or made in a factory producing nuts. Also remember that John Hopkins Medical Center warns autoimmune sufferers to avoid garlic and Echinacea supplements as these boost your immune system thus possibly making you feel worse.

Stress & Coping Techniques

Remove or reduce negative stressors from your life. Stress is known to worsen UCTD symptoms and might even trigger a flare. Stress is inevitable and how we handle stress may be a bigger determinant of our health than previously thought. Stress may be as minor as forgetting a simple task to being a major life changing occurrence. According to the MedlinePlus, part of the U.S. National Library of Medicine, stress may be routine, caused by unexpected negative factors or traumatic[57].

Routine stressors happen in our everyday lives. From daily chores, work tasks and basic family interactions, routine stressors are inevitable. This type of stress is manageable and may include creating schedules to better manage time and responsibilities. Unexpected negative stressors require more involvement and take more of a toll of a person's psyche.

Unexpected and unwanted stressors could include divorce, unemployment, major family squabbles and chronic illness. As UCTD sufferers, we live with a chronic illness that is not only a stress on our body but also on our mental and emotional health.

Traumatic stress[56] is the most destructive stress to our emotional well-being and can also impact our physical self in the worst possible way. Traumatic experiences include being involved in a major natural disaster, losing someone close to you (such as murder), living in or being a soldier in a war zone or being involved in an accident. Such traumatic experiences can have profound effect on the body.

You, like me, might have read or listened to news stories of persons becoming blind after severe or prolonged stress and may suffer from heart attacks or strokes. Stress causes more blood to pump to the heart thus raising the heart rate as well as causing hypertensive conditions in the body. According to the Mayo Clinic, stress also negatively impacts the immune system and causes a fight or flight response which may take prolonged periods of time for the body to recover[59]. The longer the body undergoes stressful situations the more likely chronic inflammation is likely to occur. This does not mean that stress is the reason for chronic inflammation but it is one of the known factors; one that can be managed.

Work & Money

For UCTD patients, we sometimes undergo long-term stressors including work concerns and money issues relating to paying our medical bills. It is astounding how quickly many of us move from being fully active to having to give up jobs we love. In some cases, when jobs terminate our services, our only source of income disappears and this serves to create a highly stressful environment.

Money is not everything (although some might disagree) but when you are sick, the true importance of money becomes apparent. In some cases, UCTD patients may not have had health insurance or maybe the insurance company dropped you because of the many claims or sometimes even with insurance, the co-pay is simply too high. Consequently, one of the most pressing issues I have encountered among persons with chronic illnesses is the stress about money.

As some persons with chronic illness lose an income, money stressors may magnify within the family. It is not unheard of to hear of subsequent divorces among married couples. Many times I have seen the question on Internet support group boards- "How do I manage now that I do not work?" You have once active persons who were nurses, teachers and other professionals being constrained to their homes.

Personally, I know that the times when I was unable to work were stressful periods. I had the knowledge and skills but could not physically manage at that time. You cannot help but to wonder where the money is coming from to cover your household and medical bills.

I do not know about anyone else, but each time I get a new prescription I begin to worry. If the doctor tells me the drug is new, I worry even more. Why, you might ask? The newer the drug, the more expensive it is. Our condition means we are normally prescribed multiple drugs and that simply means a higher bill at the pharmacy. When you start spending upwards of $150 USD and I have heard of $350 per month on medicine alone and you are NOT working, one can hardly help feeling stressed.

Is money not a stressor for you? How about all those different medical tests your doctor wants you to take? How about the cost to see a specialist? You see, in Jamaica, I can see a neurologist, my rheumatologist, my primary care physician and a gastroenterologist all for just about $280 USD and that might include change to get lunch. I am quite aware however that one visit in the USA runs about that price just to see a PCP or emergent care. As such, the cost to see the doctor can be quite prohibitive to many. So you are either stressed because you do not have the money to see the doctor, or stressed because you saw the doctor and have the bill to pay.

I recently told hubby that it is cheaper to fly to Jamaica and schedule a visit with all the different specialists as needed that to pay for it within the USA. Can you see why medical tourism is taking off in so many countries? I am not advocating you seeking foreign treatment, but I am simply adding up the costs of healthcare in a country like the USA.

Family

Family issues are another major source of stressor for persons with chronic illnesses. While healthy individuals will say that everyone has family issues, the truth is those issues are sometimes magnified in the presence of a chronic illness. Persons with chronic illnesses know firsthand the difficulty family members accepting that they are indeed ill.

For those who are unable to self-maintain themselves, the added burden of family members being caretakers, adds an additional element of stress to the family dynamics. Additionally, the UCTD patient is also apt to believe him or herself a burden on the family and this can causes the patient to stress daily on the issue.

For those UCTD with young families, the stress of managing a household especially while working can be daunting. There are no days off even when you do not feel well. The perfect storm is having kids under 10, animal(s), a home to maintain and a full-time job. While this scenario is difficult for any healthy persons, it is even more difficult for a person with an autoimmune condition. Due to pain, swelling, fatigue or other issues, it might become difficult to complete all the tasks that must be accomplished each day. This can lead to feelings of guilt and an overwhelming sense of pressure. Such pressure is simply another word for stress.

Other Factors Promoting Stress

Stress might be more predisposed in certain individuals[57]. Do you know someone who is always stressed? Stressing over even the minutest issues? Perhaps that person cannot handle stressors as well as you can. That person through personality trait, prior illness or genes might not be able to deal with stress. Some persons have what might be looked at as a run of bad luck or a series of unfortunate events. Consecutive negative events do not give an individual a chance to recover and thus causes prolonged stressors on the body.

Another cause of stress is positive life events[60]. At this point you are probably wondering how the word positive can lead to stress. Well positive life events are desirable events such as weddings, parties, special events, graduations and pregnancies. Unfortunately, these positive events are not easily identifiable as causing stress. Think of a wedding, are you the bride or groom? If so, you have millions of small details to 'worry' about. And if you are as detail-oriented as my husband, then your stress levels rise just thinking about all you have to accomplish.

Another happy event such as having a baby is a wondrous event, but not only does that bring about changes in the family dynamics and financial concerns but it also puts a toll on the mother's body. Surprisingly, some women do really well during pregnancy and even with UCTD or other autoimmune conditions, stay remarkably healthy. However, there are those women whose health conditions worsen or for whom new health issues arise during pregnancy. These women may experience as rise in their stress levels which may worsen their preexisting conditions.

Coping Strategies

One of the first ways to handle stress is by identifying your stressors. Once you have identified your stressors then you will be better able to deal with them. Identification of your stressors is also important as you will be able to discuss these stressors in your cognitive behavior therapy session (discussed below). Discussing your stressors and meeting them head-on is one way of reducing the impact of these stressors on you.

Additionally, consider small ways to cope with stress and reduce stress in your life. Consider reducing your hours at work, requesting a change in job responsibilities or changing to a less stressful job as any of these options may have beneficial effects on your health. The less stress you have at work the more likely your health will improve because of decreased stress. If you have lost your job and thus your income, try other means of sourcing an income. Check reputable online job opportunities. Turn your hobby into an income earner and sell on Etsy or eBay. Find ways to earn an alternate income and do not give up. Giving up is one of the worst things you can do for your mental health.

Sometimes your home may be the thing that is stressful as you are unable to move and lift items as you once could. With limited movement in hands and feet, the simplest tasks may seem magnified. Simple coping strategies include making your home friendly to your condition. This might require changing doorknobs that become difficult to open because of painful or weak hands. Get cabinet drawers that are easy to open and faucets that are easy to turn on. Consider levered pipes where possible and if you are renting, consider renting a home without stairs as that might minimize the pressure on your joints.

Other than these simple coping techniques previously mentioned, there are several anti-stress techniques that you may employ:

Cognitive Behavior Therapy

Some persons balk at the term cognitive behavior therapy (CBT) as they believe that only persons with mental issues and depression will require such an intervention. This psychotherapy is however, extremely useful to persons living with chronic illnesses as it provides coping mechanisms and an improved way of looking at life[61]. CBT requires meeting with a mental health counselor for predetermined sessions and during these sessions discuss ways to deal with the frustration of living with a disease. CBT does not have to include medication although anti-depressants may be used if the patient is experiencing anxiety attacks and depressive episodes.

In a CBT session, the patient discusses any fears and resentment towards the disease they have and discuss acceptance techniques to help them cope. Persons with autoimmune diseases like UCTD will find it easier to accept the disease label and reduce their stress surrounding the disease once they learn coping techniques. CBT might not work for everyone but it worth a try. I have not done formal CBT but I found self-help sites and developed my own coping techniques to help me develop a more positive outlook on my life with UCTD/Fibro.

Meditation, Tai Chi & Yoga

Meditation is the practice of focusing your thoughts in order to create a calmer mind. Sometimes the mind is jumbled and meditation is a way of clearing those thoughts by finding a quiet place to contemplate. Find a space in your house that is quiet, or choose a time of day that allows you to separate from the chaos around you. Recommendations include preparing your mind for meditation by reading suitable reflective materials. There are books or instructional guides that teach you how to meditate.

Tai chi (Ti-chi) is a gentle and graceful form of exercise involving slow movements and incorporating deep breathing. Tai-chi is a low impact exercise and is gentle enough to practice during pregnancy. Tai-chi keeps the body constantly moving but is easy on the joints and ligaments. Check out your local martial arts studio or senior citizen center for Tai-chi classes. Some cities might have Tai-chi in the park in the mornings so check your city guide or information.

Yoga is another great option to promote peacefulness and meditation while exercising the body. In the absence of a yoga class, I have used the yoga exercise on my Wii Fit as a means of both exercise and meditation. Yoga combines mind and body techniques to bring about relaxation and helps to de-stress the practitioner. Yoga includes stretching and deep breathing and is helpful in opening up the body while being gentle on the limbs.

There are various forms of yoga but at the core of the practice, is the understanding that yoga can improve strength and flexibility of the practitioner. Be careful when choosing a yoga class and ensure that the yoga practitioner is certified or trained. Furthermore, if you are hurting after doing yoga, consider speaking to your instructor. There have been cases of persons injuring themselves doing yoga poses. Although these cases seem to be few, it is advisable for persons with compromised joint functions to be careful when practicing certain poses[62].

Meditation like Tai chi and yoga has gotten a negative rap from some Christians who believe it requires worshipping another deity or opening up the mind and leaving it open to evil spirits. How do I know this? I grew up hearing this from my Christian circle. As I grew older, I realized the fallacy of that thought process and I now recognize meditation for the true benefit that it offers - peace. Of course the thoughts you focus on will be important. If you are Christian-minded and bothered by the thoughts of Eastern philosophies, focus your thoughts on bible texts or Christian literature to center yourself while meditating.

Diet – Eating the Right Foods

Nutrition is important to the UCTD patient. Unfortunately, the nutritional intake of UCTD patients may not be ideal and might actually contribute to the patient's ill health. Some UCTD patients may not even recognize that the food they eat could be a trigger or a contributor to their suffering. Food sensitivity is now a recognized issue with autoimmune patients and you may find increasing numbers of information from reputable medical centers like John Hopkins publishing literature on how to avoid food sensitivities and triggers.

The degree of food sensitivities vary from person to person. In some cases, UCTD patients may not be aware of their sensitivities to certain type of foods. Eating these foods can cause either an immediate or delayed reaction on the body resulting in increased inflammation or other negative body reactions. Literature on foods sensitivities normally will center on the main culprits - gluten (wheat), soy, dairy, corn and nuts although persons may also react to other food ingredients.

Please understand that each autoimmune disease might have its own set of triggers and so no single autoimmune dietary recommendation might address the issues of every single disease. Persons suffering from Celiac disease will have a stronger negative reaction to gluten than maybe a patient with UCTD. It is faulty to assume that because both diseases are autoimmune then the triggers must be the same.

When reading materials advocating information on foods to avoid or eat, consider if the information has any scientific basis or is it simply the ideas of an individual. I believe in both science and tried and true home remedies, however I am cautious about any information that does not seem to have a strong basis in facts. I am even more troubled if the recommendation seems a way to get me to buy some new super vitamin or super food that no other company has. And if the material starts telling me of a cure-all product or lifestyle, personally, I stop reading. Again, it is your life and you will have to make decisions on whose advice to follow.

Your food choices might be affected by your current mindset. Do you follow the alarmists who believe every food is designed to kill them? Those that believe that fruits and real fruit juices are bad, water must be alkaline and without live active cultures in your diet you cannot do well. Or do you lean to the findings of new scientific studies that were backed by pharmaceutical companies? Can you trust such studies?

My general recommendation is to do your own research and do not rely on only one study, book or website for your information. Understand that no matter how publicized a study finding's, it may not be generalizable to the general population. Hence, you must be prepared to look beyond the sensationalist headlines of the newspapers, the news anchors and authors.

Specific Anti Inflammatory Diets

Dr. White who is the chief public health officer at the US Arthritis Foundation postulated that diet may not have the intended benefits on arthritic conditions as originally thought[63]. She noted that current studies do not provide enough proof to draw that conclusion. Elisa Zied, a registered dietician with American Dietetic Association noted that the focus should be on the overall nutrition rather than specific anti-inflammatory diets[63]. Nonetheless patients do anecdotally report successes following these diets.

Gluten-free Diet

As discussed in chapter 2, some autoimmune conditions like Celiac disease are triggered by gluten (primarily in wheat based products). Such persons must avoid gluten if they are to feel well. Other persons have realized that they feel better without gluten in their diet and report gaining more energy and less negative symptoms. If there is a true allergy or intolerance to gluten the person would have Celiac disease, otherwise the person will most likely suffer from gluten sensitivities. Being sensitive to gluten is not the same as being allergic or intolerant to gluten. This distinction is important as adopting a gluten-free lifestyle does not mean it will make every person following the diet feel better.

A gluten-free (GF) lifestyle means adjusting the diet to eliminate ALL traces of gluten. Outside of the obvious, wheat, barley & rye products, gluten is sometimes hidden in our foods- sauces, gravies, salad dressings, soy sauce, pill casings, just to name a few. This diet requires commitment and may be very beneficial to some autoimmune sufferers even if they do not suffer from Celiac. You can test for gluten allergies but you must be eating gluten in order to do the test.

With the increase in numbers of persons following the GF lifestyle, there are more GF food options available in the supermarkets. New GF cookbooks are published daily and these offer persons the opportunity to create exciting and tasty dishes that do not require gluten ingredients. Consider also following blogs dedicated to the GF lifestyle for tips and tricks on how to maintain a GF lifestyle such as places to eat out and substitute ingredients to stock.

Notwithstanding the benefits of a GF lifestyle for some, in my humble estimation, for some persons, GF is the new fad diet. A GF diet can be very restrictive and I know persons who have begun the diet and stopped due to the limitations and cost of the diet. This diet therefore is not as simple as replacing bread and flours. Going gluten free means relearning to stock your panty with gluten-free alternatives and making gluten free dishes.

Persons leading a GF lifestyle must also be careful to maintain a balanced diet as the GF diet removes whole grains (fiber) and by extension some vitamins and minerals[64]. Another concern is that the replacement GF foods are often high in sugar and low in fiber. Persons on the GF diet must therefore ensure that they add enough fiber in their diet and take additional vitamins and supplements if they are to remain healthy.

Paleo Diet

Similar to the Atkins diet, in terms of the low carb approach, the Paleo diet attempts to replicate the diet of our prehistoric ancestors. The premise of the diet is that by eating like our "cavemen" ancestors we will be leaner and less prone to developing lifestyle diseases like cancer, heart problems and diabetes. The Paleo diet advocates less processed foods and replacing the diet with wholesome foods. The diet also recommends consuming leaner cuts of meat and reducing refined fats. Proponents of the Paleo diet also tout adding fruits, vegetables, seeds and nuts as well as eggs in order to create a balanced diet.

One of the main benefits of the Paleo diet to autoimmune sufferers like UCTD patients is that it eliminates all grains including wheat and wheat related grains. In the absence of gluten, some patients may see a definite improvement in their symptoms. Additionally, consuming wholesome foods such as grass-fed meats, organically grown fruits and vegetables should undoubtedly result in a more healthy body.

Critics of the Paleo diet seemingly doubt the effectiveness of the diet given the fact that the diet eliminates grains (fiber) and legumes (beans & peas); foods that some consider essential parts of the food pyramid. Other foods excluded from the diet are dairy, refined sugars, salt and potatoes. Interestingly, you might notice that the list of excluded foods seem to be the ones that are most vilified as likely to trigger autoimmune conditions. Critics also worry that Paleo practitioners may be missing essential vitamins and minerals due to their elimination of grains and dairy.

On personal reflection, I think this diet is worth considering. I may doubt and disagree with the hunter-gatherer premise of the Paleo diet, but I can see potential benefits in attempting it. If you have not had much luck with medications and supplements eliminating or reducing your symptoms, maybe you too could research further, the Paleo diet to see if would work for you.

General Anti-Inflammatory Diet

For persons who believe that foods can help or worsen their autoimmune conditions but do not want a restrictive diet, then they can consider a general anti-inflammatory diet. This diet does not eliminate grains or meats or fats. Persons following this diet are more likely to favor whole foods and eschew processed foods.

Recent concerns on food safety and genetically modified foods (GMO) have created a burgeoning whole foods industry. As more persons try to eat healthier, the demand for organically produced foods has skyrocketed. Persons are realizing that more thought must be given to the food they eat and that involves being aware of ingredients in the foods they consume.

Recently, as I stood in the supermarket about to purchase a no-cholesterol spread, I happened to glance over at the butter. Bear in mind I had not purchased butter since about 2007. Like many others, I use light margarine spreads in lieu of butter. I too, had become convinced that butter was full of saturated fats and therefore bad for me.

Eight years later, as I look at the ingredient list of both products, I realize that the list of ingredients on the spread includes ingredients I cannot pronounce and does include the dreaded partially hydrogenated oil. Glancing over at the salted butter, I note two ingredients, cream and salt. Right there I had a ha-ha moment; a pivotal shift in my grocery list mindset.

I began remembering as a child in Jamaica where coconut oil was king and everyone cooked with it. Then came all the studies and experts touting with alacrity how bad coconut oil was for our health. Bye bye coconut oil and welcome hydrogenated vegetable oil, soy oil and GMO corn oil. I therefore find it almost amusing that experts are once again touting how great coconut oil is; albeit this time around, the price of coconut oil has skyrocketed out of reach of typical consumers.

These recent experiences made me re-examine the way I was making my decision to purchase foods. In trying to lose weight and be healthy, I had swapped real foods for plastic sounding ingredients. Why had I changed my diet? How had I gotten sucked into the food hype? After all, my father at 85 years old eats the most sugar, oil, gravy and salt and has only since 2013 started experiencing mild arthritic pains.

At my dad's age, his cholesterol is good, blood pressure 110/65, no diabetes and no other lifestyle illnesses. Now as my father notes, he smoked in his younger years. He grew up poor and his diet included eating condensed milk on bread, eating wet sugar as well as eating heavy carbohydrate laden meals. How then did he remain well? Could it be that the unprocessed foods he used to eat were a contributing factor? I cannot dismiss genetic coding as playing a role in my dad's health, but given that all his older children have hypertension among other issues, there might be more to his food history that helps explain the importance of the foods we eat.

In no way am I using my dad's story as the end-all, know-all, but it is an anecdotal representation of yesteryear where people ate real foods. If real foods fortify our bodies, then maybe it is time to rethink our shopping lists. Why not start by substituting products that have too long an ingredient list or the names are too difficult to pronounce. Remember that food companies often hide ingredients in plain sight by listing the scientific name; one that you would never reconcile with the commonly accepted name.

Many persons seeking better health are trying to follow a clean diet. For those trying to eat clean, here are some quick tips for following an anti-inflammatory diet:

Research the foods you eat. For example, who says butter is bad for you and that margarine is superior?[65] Are those studies still relevant? Remember studies age and new studies and emerging information occur every day. Fascinatingly, did you know that the trans-fat in margarine can be worse for your heart than the saturated fats in butter?

If you must use fats, it would be better to use olive oil than either butter or margarine and remember to use oils sparingly. Bake, broil or grill instead of fry. Use avocado, applesauce, sour cream or non-fat plain yogurt in baking your cakes instead of oil or butter. Did you know that ground flaxseed can be used as a substitute for fats like butter or even for eggs in your recipes? Why not substitute some ground flaxseed the next time you are baking or add to your smoothie or oatmeal.

Drink lots of water - it is better to drink purified water and some suggest alkaline water. The body simply requires clean water but you can choose the type of water you consume. Try to consume pure water without additives and colorings.

Avoid refined food and additives – choose whole food or refined foods. Opt for brown flour and brown rice over white flour and white rice. Cook foods from scratch rather than purchasing pre-packaged meals that contain

109

preservatives and additives. The fresher the ingredient, the better it is for the health of your body. I can attest to serving up tastier foods when I cook at home and saving money in the process. The cost of eating out for two persons three nights per week at even the most basic quick service restaurant can set us back $100 (including tax & tip). And that's with drinking water. For the same $100 I can feed us for a week.

Add Omega 3 fatty acids – eat wild salmon and mackerel over farm-raised. The beautiful pink could be as a result of additives. Wild caught salmon although more expensive, is a better option. Also consider quality fish oils and use Krill oil where possible. Walnut is also a great non-meat option that provides omega 3.

Choose organic meats from range free animals – as much as possible stick to lean cuts of meat. Buy organic meats where possible and minimize consumption of red meat.

Eat whole grains – whole grains are better for your diet. Whole grains are superior to refined grain as they retain their bran and germ. Whole grains are great sources of fiber. Do not confuse enriched grains with whole grains. Enriched grains have added vitamin B but with none of the benefits of the fiber found in whole grains.

Do not be fooled by the ads and hype on some cereal boxes. Buy your grains whole and cook yourself. Recipes abound online on how to make your own cereal and muesli. If you eat grains, consider whole grains instead of stripped grains. Choose steel cut oats over instant oats. Switch white rice for brown or wild rice and if not allergic to gluten, add bulgur wheat for fiber.

Increase your fruits and vegetable consumption - fresh fruits and vegetable can provide fiber and natural vitamins. Some of these vitamins are great in helping to build a healthier body.

Elimination Diet

The elimination diet involves removing certain foods from your diet. The belief is that some foods are detrimental to your health and is the cause of your illness. Common culprits include gluten, night shade vegetables and sugar. Gluten is often one of the first things person tries to eliminate from their diet. You may eliminate gluten from your diet for a while and see if your symptoms improve. If they do, then you might consider going GF. On the other hand, if you saw no noticeable change, then going permanently GF might not yield much benefit.

Nightshade vegetables have gotten a bad rap and even in the absence of irrefutable research, been blamed for contributing to inflammation[66]. Nightshade vegetables include sweet peppers, tomatoes, potatoes and eggplants. Eliminating all nightshade vegetables might still be a good idea in testing to see if they aggravate your condition. Alternately, you may eliminate each nightshade vegetable at a time to see if it is only one or all that is triggering your illness.

Personally, I have found that nightshades do not make me worse or better. I have eliminated them and then reintroduced them and have seen no difference in my pain or swelling levels. As such, I do not subscribe to nightshade vegetables being harmful to my health.

Sugar has come under increasing pressure from health advocates as to its damaging effects on the body. Sugar is known as the sweet poison and in order to feel better, it is advisable to reduce your intake of sugar laden and carbohydrate dense foods. According to a Harvard Medical School Family Health Guide, eating too much sugar increases level of cytokines which is a known inflammation messenger[67]. Sugar has been known to increase inflammation or worsen inflammation issues thus aggravating autoimmune issues.

I know there are those who say to just stop eating sugar, but from my experience and observing persons around me who have tried, I can categorically state that this method is more likely to fail. Once persons go on a very restrictive diet, it seems that there seems to be a point where they give up and go back to eating sugar as normal. I ask you to examine yourself and see if eliminating sugar is something that you can do and maintain. If the answer is yes, then this might be the best option for you.

For those who cannot give up sugar easily, please do not feel defeated; you are probably in the majority of persons who have not been able to ditch sugar in totality. Do not feel brow beaten because you couldn't do it in one fell swoop. One of the easiest ways persons find to give up sugar is by substituting sweeteners like Splenda and Aspartame[68].

In recent times, you might have seen increasing concern about these two sweeteners. Splenda is said to affect the neurological functions of the body and for autoimmune patients who already might have neuropathy issues, this would not be a positive. Aspartame I KNOW firsthand triggers my joint pains. Aspartame is suspected to be carcinogenic to humans despite the US FDA refuting such claims.

If you are unsure about any food entering your mouth then I would advise elimination of such foods. If you chose to eliminate artificial sweeteners, that would be mean avoiding many diet and light (lite) drinks that reduce calories by removing sugar and replacing with these artificial sweeteners. If you cannot use the sweeteners you are used to as they might make you sick, what are your other options in order for you to give up sugar? Consider the options below:

Natural sweeteners

Find natural alternatives to your existing artificial sweeteners. Monk fruit is a lower glycemic index sweetener that is lower in calorie than sugar and does not have the negative side effects of both sugar and the artificial alternatives. Persons also substitute Agave nectar, honey and molasses but the reality is that the body more or less might react to these sweeteners in the same way as sugar.

Reduce your natural sugar inclinations

If you used to use 4 tablespoons, try to use 3 tablespoons and gradually try to trick your taste buds into taking in less sugar.

In replacing drinks, add fruit slices and create your own fruit water by infusing the fruit flavor without the added sugar. Try infusions such as mint & cucumber, strawberry & lemon, mint & lemon and triple berry (blackberry, raspberry & blueberry) infusions.

Swap bad sugars for good sugars

The next time your reach for a piece of cake think which fruit could you have substituted it with. Replace ice cream with frozen pureed mango or strawberry. Replace cake with a fruit salad and top with fresh cream (if not lactose intolerant). While fruits contain sugar, the sugar in fruits will be a better option that carbohydrate heavy pastries and frozen desserts.

The Role of Prayer & Faith

As a Christian, I believe in prayer and my faith has helped me through many a dark time[69]. Increasingly, the medical community is paying attention to the role of prayer in a patient's life and recovery from illness and surgery. Once shunned by the medical society, studies have been commissioned on the role of prayer on the healing of patients. According to WebMD, one such study commissioned by the NIH and funded by the US Congress, seeks to understand how prayer impacts the health of a patient[70].

For those who are not Christians, understand that you will need to find your own faith-centered or belief-anchored crutch to lean on during your health crisis. The four-page

WebMD article does note that that health benefits are also possible from centering on Buddhist prayers or any repetitive meditation designed to center you. . Please feel free to skip this section if you do not wish to read further on the impact of faith and prayer during your illness (one reason why I placed it at the back of the book).

The article also provides information on research that tentatively shows that persons who are religious and spiritually active are less likely to become depressed or remain depressed. This reminded me of a conversation with my friend who is a doctor in Canada. She shared with me anecdotally that she noticed that her religious patients were less likely to request or need anti-depressants. She found that they were more likely to tell her they would pray or depend on God for strength rather than depend on medication.

Like those persons, I too can attest to my faith bringing me through periods of chemically induced anxiety attacks. Depending on the medication(s) I take, I sometimes have the unfortunate side effect of anxiety. In one particular case, it was so bad that it was keeping me up every night. Every sound around the house had my heart racing and I would curl into ball wishing morning light to alleviate the unwanted anxiety.

To deal with my anxiety, instead of taking antidepressants, I chose to reach for my bible and used bible texts to anchor me and fortify me. There is a particular text found in 2 Timothy, 1 verse 7 – "For God hath not given us the spirit of fear; but of power, and of love, and of a sound mind." I read this and used it as a mantra each night and would fall asleep peacefully despite the underlying anxiety. In short order, about 5 nights of doing this, and my anxiety waned. I could feel it, but it was no longer a pressing issue. I believed that the anxiety wouldn't win, and it did not.

There has been times however where not even my faith could sustain me. I had to abruptly stop taking prednisone for my UCTD symptoms and Cymbalta for my Fibromyalgia back pain as I had severe gastrointestinal disturbances. Normally, you should be weaned off the prednisone and Cymbalta, but I stopped cold turkey. I experienced the worst feeling of rage and anger and could not shake the feeling on my own.

Even with prayer and my trusty bible text, I had to end up seeing a doctor. The doctor prescribed me with antidepressants to help me through the withdrawal stage of the Cymbalta. Instead of taking the pill for a month and filling the repeat, I took it for two weeks as that was all I needed as a crutch.

Despite my firm belief in prayer and healing, I have an issue with what I perceive as a growing trend among some Christians. This practice of faith healing that through the laying of hands and the claim that faith alone can heal you raises many issues with me. All Christians know they can pray for healing, but I am concerned when a person who is ill tells me they are ill because their church/other members tell them they haven't prayed or believed enough.

I have been on the receiving end of that logic when a new hairdresser told me that I didn't really want to be well or I would have the faith to wish myself well. Another told me that her back used to hurt but she simply prayed it away. And while I believe in miracles and healing, I wonder which bible such persons are reading that I haven't read.

I have read wonderful stories of miraculous healings but also noted that many of those persons suffered for years; their healing wasn't instantaneous. In some cases, even the beloved and chosen like Paul (St. Paul) suffered and yet God said "My grace is sufficient." If I have learnt nothing else in bible study it is that God answers in different ways; he heals immediately, he makes you to wait or he lets you know that it is your burden to bear.

As such, my ire is with ludicrous persons who persist in noting that illness is due to a lack of faith. Furthermore, I know so many good persons with extremely strong faith who have died. Some even were successful in praying for others to receive healing. How then did some of these people die from illness? Why did some of them suffer before death? Was that a lack of their faith? Or was it just the scheme of things?

I am not professing to have the biblical or spiritual answers. I am simply showing how during my UCTD journey I have suffered even at the hands of those who professed to be doing something good for my spirituality. On a spiritual plane I have come to a place of acceptance of my illness. As long as I dwelt on miraculous healing it left me prone to thoughts of not being holy enough or worthy enough as to why I wasn't healed. However, at this point in my life, I pray for healing and recovery but have developed the faith to accept if it doesn't come.

I am a realist, I am practical and I live in the here and now. I believe in the absence of healing that doctors exist to provide medical intervention. I am not against taking medications if it means getting well but I would love to stop taking them. Please do not let anyone convince you to give up medication as your proof that you have faith. If you believe in God and His omnipotence, understand that God can heal you even if you are taking medication. What kind of small box some must put God in if they believe that he will only heal if you opt out of medical care.

I have seen too many news reports about children who died from simple illnesses as their parent waited on divine intervention. I also know first-hand accounts of persons who stopped taking medication because their pastor or preacher told them to. Those reports reminded me of a well-known story about the man who was drowning who rejected numerous offers of help because he was waiting on God to rescue him. The man died and went to heaven and asked God why He didn't rescue him to which God replied, "I sent you rescuers, but your rejected them all."

Looking Ahead

Despite your best efforts, you might find that the disease refuses to release its stranglehold on you. I admonish you to keep trying. Sometimes a technique might be successful the second time around. Remain upbeat and surround yourself with positive people. Eliminate all negativity from your life. Call on your faith, - we all have one. Where does your faith lie? Discover the strong person within and despite all your health challenges, do not be afraid to let that person shine.

I wish for all you my readers, improved health, wellness and peace of mind.

THE END

AUTHOR'S NOTE

Thank you for having purchased this book and I hope this book has proved helpful to you. You will find sufficient references with corresponding links that might provide you with even deeper insights into autoimmune conditions. I hope that through your own research, you will develop the tools necessary to help chart your course to good health.

I would love to hear from you. Please feel free to share both your comments and criticisms. Please visit my site at http://www.kimberlymcbee.com if you need to contact me or discuss any information provided in this book. I thank your for your time and for having purchased this book. Where possible, please leave a review of the book as it may be helpful for others who are searching for a book about UCTD.

OTHER BOOKS BY THE AUTHOR

Available online on Amazon and other fine retailers

How to Cook Jamaican Cookbook 1: Authentic Fish & Meat Recipes (The Back to the Kitchen Cookbook Series)

How to Cook Jamaican Cookbook 2: Traditional Salads, Sides & Starters (The Back to the Kitchen Cookbook Series)

How to Cook Jamaican Cookbook 3: Sumptuous Porridge & Soup Recipes (The Back to the Kitchen Cookbook Series)

Coming Soon:

How to Cook Jamaican Cookbook 4: Yummy Desserts, Drinks & Cocktails (The Back to the Kitchen Cookbook Series)

ONLINE SUPPORT GROUPS

A list of some online support groups:

Daily Strength

http://www.dailystrength.org/c/MCTD/support-group

Facebook

https://www.facebook.com/groups/UCTDsupportgroup/

https://www.facebook.com/groups/Autoimmunerealtimesu
pport/?ref=br_rs

Healing Well

http://www.healingwell.com/community/default.aspx?c=4

Healthboards

http://www.healthboards.com/boards/#immune-
autoimmune

I make no recommendation about these support groups. I am only providing a limited list of the ones that I know are active groups at the time of publication. Feel free to browse the support groups and join the one best suited to your needs.

REFERENCES

1. Berman, J.R. (2003) Undifferentiated Connective Tissue Disease - In-Depth Overview. Retrieved November 26, 2013 from http://www.hss.edu/conditions_undifferentiated-connective-tissue-disease-overview.asp

2. Undifferentiated Connective Tissue Disease (UCTD): Frequently Asked Questions (2004). Retrieved November 26, 2013 from http://www.hss.edu/conditions_undifferentiated-connective-tissue-disease-faqs.asp

3. Undifferentiated Connective Tissue Disease (UCTD): Overview (2013). Retrieved November 26, 2013 from http://www.nationaljewish.org/healthinfo/conditions/uctd/

4. Undifferentiated Connective Tissue Disease Case: Distinct Clinical Entity?: Discussion of Diagnosis (2008). Retrieved November 26, 2013 from http://www.medscape.org/viewarticle/572828_3

5. Mixed Connective Tissue Disease. (2012). Retrieved November 28, 2013 from http://www.mayoclinic.com/health/mixed-connective-tissue-disease/DS00675

6. What is an inflammation? (2011). PubMed Health. Retrieved November 28, 2013 from http://www.ncbi.nlm.nih.gov/pubmedhealth/PMH0009852/

7. The Immune System - in More Detail. (2013). Nobelprize.org. Retrieved December 19 from http://www.nobelprize.org/educational/medicine/immunity/immune-detail.html

8. ANA Test (2011). Mayo Clinic. Retrieved January 23, 2014 from http://www.mayoclinic.org/tests-procedures/ana-test/basics/definition/prc-20014566

9. Fairweather D, Rose NR. Women and autoimmune diseases. Emerg Infect Dis v.10(11) doi: 10.3201/eid1011.040367. Retrieved December 19, 2013 from http://www.ncbi.nlm.nih.gov/pmc/articles/PMC3328995/

10. Undifferentiated Connective Tissue Disease (UCTD): Frequently Asked Questions. (2009). Hospital for Special Surgery. Retrieved November 26, 2013 from http://www.hss.edu/conditions_undifferentiated-connective-tissue-disease-faqs.asp

11. Undifferentiated Connective Tissue Disease (UCTD): Symptoms (2013). Retrieved November 26, 2013 from http://www.nationaljewish.org/healthinfo/conditions/uctd/symptoms/

12. Peripheral neuropathy. (2013). Retrieved November 28, 2013 from http://www.mayoclinic.com/health/peripheral-neuropathy/DS00131

13. Vann, M. (2009).Vision Problems and Autoimmune Disorders. Retrieved November 21, 2013 from http://www.everydayhealth.com/autoimmune-

disorders/vision-problems-and-autoimmune-disorders.aspx

14. Fever (n.d.). The Ohio State Ohio University- Wexner Medical Center. Retrieved November 21, 2013 from http://medicalcenter.osu.edu/patientcare/healthcare_serv ices/pediatrics/common_childhood_illness/infections/fe vers/Pages/index.aspx

15. Joint Pain. (2013). Retrieved November 21, 2013 from http://www.mayoclinic.com/health/joint-pain/MY00187

16. Mosca, M., Tani, C., Carli, L. & Bombardier, S. (2012). Undifferentiated CTD: A Wide Spectrum of Autoimmune Diseases. Best Practice & Research Clinical Rheumatology 26 (2012) 73–77 doi:10.1016/j.berh.2012.01.005 Retrieved December 16, 2013 from http://211.144.68.84:9998/91keshi/Public/File/12/26-1/pdf/1-s2.0-S152169421200006X-main.pdf.

17. Connective Tissue Diseases. (2011). The Cleveland Clinic. Retrieved November 28, 2013 from http://my.clevelandclinic.org/disorders/connective-tissue-diseases/hic-connective-tissue-diseases.aspx

18. Understanding Scleroderma. (n.d.). The John Hopkins Scleroderma Centre. Retrieved November 24, 2013 from http://www.hopkinsscleroderma.org/scleroderma/

19. Polymyositis-and-Dermatomyositis. (2014). Cedars-Sinai. Retrieved January 23, 2014 from http://www.cedars-sinai.edu/Patients/Health-Conditions/Polymyositis-and-Dermatomyositis.aspx

20. Lyme Disease. (2012). Retrieved November 21, 2013 from http://www.mayoclinic.com/health/lyme-disease/DS00116/DSECTION=symptoms

21. Sickle Cell Anemia. (2011). Retrieved November 21, 2013 from http://www.mayoclinic.com/health/sickle-cell-anemia/DS00324/DSECTION=symptoms

22. What is Crohn's Disease? (2013). Crohn's & Colitis Foundation of America. Retrieved November 21, 2013 from http://www.ccfa.org/what-are-crohns-and-colitis/what-is-crohns-disease/

23. Celiac Disease. (2013). Retrieved November 21, 2013 from http://www.mayoclinic.com/health/celiac-disease/DS00319

24. Understanding Thyroid Problems—the Basics. (2013). Women's Health. Retrieved November 28, 2013 from http://women.webmd.com/guide/understanding-thyroid-problems-basics

25. Hypothyroidism (underactive thyroid). (2012). Retrieved November 28, 2013 from http://www.mayoclinic.com/health/hypothyroidism/DS00353/DSECTION=symptoms

26. Hyperthyroidism (overactive thyroid). (2012). Retrieved November 28, 2013 from http://www.mayoclinic.com/health/hyperthyroidism/DS00344

27. Signs, Symptoms, and Co-occuring Conditions. (n.d.). The John Hopkins Lupus Centre. Retrieved December 15, 2013 from http://www.hopkinslupus.org/lupus-info/lupus-signs-symptoms-comorbidities/

28. Fibromyalgia misconceptions: Interview with a Mayo Clinic expert. (2013). Fibromyalgia. Retrieved November 28, 2013 from http://www.mayoclinic.com/health/fibromyalgia/AR000 56

29. Symptoms of Chronic Fatigue Syndrome. (2013). Retrieved November 28, 2013 from http://www.nhs.uk/Conditions/Chronic-fatigue-syndrome/Pages/Symptoms.aspx

30. Fibromyalgia (FMS). (n.d.). Retrieved November 28, 2013 from http://www.sclero.org/medical/symptoms/associated/fib romyalgia/a-to-z.html

31. Fibromyalgia & Fatigue. (n.d.). Retrieved November 28, 2013 from http://www.webmd.com/fibromyalgia/guide/fibromyalgi a-and-fatigue

32. The Effects of Stress on Your Body. (2012). Retrieved January 14, 2014 from http://www.webmd.com/mental-health/effects-of-stress-on-your-body

33. Castro,C. & Gourley, M. (2010). The Journal of Allergy and Clinical Immunology vol.125, Issue 2, Supplement 2, pp. S238-S247, DOI: 10.1016/j.jaci.2009.09.041 Retrieved December 12, 2013 from http://www.ncbi.nlm.nih.gov/pmc/articles/PMC2832720 /

34. Antinuclear Antibodies (ANA). (2012). American College of Rheumatology. Retrieved January 23, 2014 from http://www.rheumatology.org/Practice/Clinical/Patients

/Diseases_And_Conditions/Antinuclear_Antibodies_(AN
A)/

35. Sed rate (erythrocyte sedimentation rate). (2013). Retrieved
    December 12, 2013 from
    http://www.mayoclinic.com/health/sed-rate/MY00343

36. Saar,P. Hermann, W. & Müller-Ladner, U. (2006)
    Rheumatology. Oxford Journals 45 (suppl 3): iii30-
    iii32.doi: 10.1093/rheumatology/kel288 Retrieved
    December 12, 2013 from
    http://rheumatology.oxfordjournals.org/content/45/sup
    pl_3/iii30.full#ref-list-1

37. Eye Doctors: Optometrists and Ophthalmologists. 2013).
    Retrieved December 12, 2013 from
    http://www.webmd.com/eye-health/eye-doctors-
    optometrists-ophthalmologists

38. Nuerology.(n.d.) Royal College of Physicians. Retrieved
    December 12, 2013 from
    http://www.rcplondon.ac.uk/specialty/neurology

39. What is a Rheumatologist? (2012). American College of
    Rheumatology. Retrieved December 12, 2013 from
    http://www.rheumatology.org/Practice/Clinical/Patients
    /What_is_a_Rheumatologist_/

40. Williams, T.J. (1978). The Role of Prostaglandins In
    Inflammation. Department of Pharmacology, Royal
    College of Surgeons of England. Retrieved December 15,
    2013 from
    http://www.ncbi.nlm.nih.gov/pmc/articles/PMC2492079
    /pdf/annrcse01488-0031.pdf

41. NSAIDs: Nonsteroidal Anti-inflammatory Drugs. (2012). American College of Rheumatologist. Retrieved December 15, 2013 from http://www.rheumatology.org/Practice/Clinical/Patients/Medications/NSAIDs__Nonsteroidal_Anti-inflammatory_Drugs/

42. Proton-Pump Inhibitors (2011). Harvard Health Publications.Harvard Medical School. Retrieved December 15, 2013 from http://www.health.harvard.edu/newsletters/Harvard_Health_Letter/2011/April/proton-pump-inhibitors

43. Disease-modifying anti-rheumatic drugs (DMARDs). (n.d). Arthritis Research UK. Retrieved December 15, 2013 from http://www.arthritisresearchuk.org/arthritis-information/drugs/dmards.aspx

44. Treating Rheumatoid Arthritis with Disease-Modifying Drugs (DMARDs) (n.d.). Rheumatoid Arthritis Health Center. Retrieved December 15, 2013 from http://www.webmd.com/rheumatoid-arthritis/guide/dmard-rheumatoid-arthritis-treatment

45. Steroids to Treat Arthritis (n.d.). Rheumatoid Arthritis Health Center. Retrieved December 15, 2013 from http://www.webmd.com/rheumatoid-arthritis/guide/steroids-to-treat-arthritis

46. Things to Avoid (n.d.). The John Hopkins Lupus Centre. Retrieved December 15, 2013 from http://www.hopkinslupus.org/lupus-info/lifestyle-additional-information/avoid/

47. Guidelines for the Diagnosis and Treatment of Fibromyalgia. (n.d.). UW Medicine Orthopaedic and

Sports Medicine. Retrieved December 15, 2013
http://www.orthop.washington.edu/?q=patient-care/articles/arthritis/guidelines-for-the-diagnosis-and-treatment-of-fibromyalgia.html

48. Exercises for Lupus (2011). Community TV: Speaking of Lupus With Christine Miserandino. Retrieved December 15, 2013 from
http://www.webmd.com/lupus/community-tv-lupus-11/lupus-exercise?page=2

49. Vitamin D. (2012). The Mayo Clinic. Retrieved December 15, 2013 from
http://www.mayoclinic.com/health/vitamin-d/NS_patient-vitamind/DSECTION=dosing

50. Vitamin D. (2011). National Institutes of Health. Retrieved December 15, 2013 from
http://ods.od.nih.gov/factsheets/VitaminD-HealthProfessional/

51. Miserandino, C. (n.d.). But You Don't Look Sick. Retrieved November 28, 2013 from
http://www.butyoudontlooksick.com/wpress/articles/written-by-christine/the-spoon-theory/

52. Wong-Baker Faces Foundation. (1983). Retrieved December 17, 2013 from
http://www.wongbakerfaces.org/

53. Pain Types and Classifications. (2013). WebMD. Retrieved December 17, 2013 from http://www.webmd.com/pain-management/guide/pain-types-and-classifications

54. Whitten, C.E.,Donovan, M. &Cristobal, K. (2005). 9(4): 9–18. Retrieved December 17, 2013 from

http://www.ncbi.nlm.nih.gov/pmc/articles/PMC3396104
/

55. Biofeedback: Using your mind to improve your health. (2013). The Mayo Clinic. Retrieved December 15, 2013 from http://www.mayoclinic.com/health/biofeedback/MY010 72

56. Acupuncture. (2012). National Health Service. Retrieved December 17, 2013 from http://www.nhs.uk/conditions/acupuncture/Pages/Intro duction.aspx

57. Stress. (2014). National Institutes of Health. Retrieved January 24, 2014 from http://www.nlm.nih.gov/medlineplus/stress.html

58. Stress. (2013). University of Maryland Medical Center. Retrieved January 10, 2014 from http://umm.edu/health/medical/reports/articles/stress

59. Stress Basics. (2011). The Mayo Clinic. Retrieved January 24, 2014 from http://www.mayoclinic.org/healthy-living/stress-management/basics/stress-basics/hlv-20049495

60. Stress Relief. (2011). The Mayo Clinic. Retrieved January 24, 2014 from http://www.mayoclinic.org/healthy-living/stress-management/basics/stress-relief/hlv-20049495

61. Cognitive behavioral therapy. (2013). Mayo clinic. Retrieved December 16, 2013 from http://www.mayoclinic.com/health/cognitive-behavioral-therapy/MY00194

62. Broad, W, J. (2013).Women's Flexibility Is a Liability (in Yoga). The New York Times Sunday Review. Retrieved December 15, 2013 from http://www.nytimes.com/2013/11/03/sunday-review/womens-flexibility-is-a-liability-in-yoga.html?_r=0

63. Anti-inflammatory Diet: Road to Good Health? (2008). Retrieved December 15, 2013 from http://www.webmd.com/food-recipes/features/anti-inflammatory-diet-road-to-good-health?page=3

64. Can a gluten-free diet help your psoriasis? (2012). National Psoriasis Foundation USA. Retrieved December 15, 2013 from   http://www.psoriasis.org/about-psoriasis/treatments/alternative/gluten-free-diet

65. Butter vs. Margarine. (2006). Harvard Health Publications. Retrieved December 15, 2013 from http://www.health.harvard.edu/healthbeat/HEALTHbeat_062106.htm

66. Jamieson-Petonic, A. (2012). Foods that Fight Inflammation—And Why You Need Them. Retrieved December 15, 2013 from http://my.clevelandclinic.org/multimedia/transcripts/1395_foods-that-fight-inflammation-and-why-you-need-them.aspx

67. What you eat can fuel or cool inflammation, a key driver of heart disease, diabetes, and other chronic conditions. (2007). Harvard Medical School family Health Guide. Retrieved December 15, 2013 from http://www.health.harvard.edu/fhg/updates/What-you-eat-can-fuel-or-cool-inflammation-a-key-driver-of-heart-disease-diabetes-and-other-chronic-conditions.shtml

68. View the Evidence: Problem Substances. (n.d.). Retrieved December 15, 2013 from http://www.greenmedinfo.com/toxic-ingredient/aspartame

69. Andrade, C. & Radhakrishnan, R. (2009). Prayer and healing: A medical and scientific perspective on randomized controlled trials. Indian Journal of Psychiatry. 2009 Oct-Dec; 51(4): 247–253. doi: 10.4103/0019-5545.58288. Retrieved January 23, 2014 from http://www.ncbi.nlm.nih.gov/pmc/articles/PMC2802370/

70. Davis, J.L. (n.d.). Can Prayer Heal? Retrieved January 23, 2014 from http://www.webmd.com/balance/features/can-prayer-heal?page=2

INDEX

Printed in Great Britain
by Amazon